PRAISE FOR *SOUL-HAPPY*

"Anette's story is an empowering example of what we can overcome when we redefine what true healing and living means."

—Amy B. Scher, author of *This is How I Save My Life* and the How to Heal series

"The strength of this work is Nilsson's presence, her voice, her honesty, and her wisdom. She's a gifted writer who has been to the edge and lived to tell about it. Reading her memoir is like reading a novel of courage and survival."

—Bonnie Hearn Hill, author of *If Anything Should Happen* and *Presumed Guilty*

"With penetrating candor and searing insight, Anette Nilsson, a gifted writer, explores her profound experience of self-denial, illness, loss, and grief as an entry point into understanding the breakdown of her own life and body . . . a raw and real read through Nilsson's journey of being broken open to uncover the ways in which truth heals and love and forgiveness can be received."

—Bridgitte Jackson-Buckley, author of *The Gift of Crisis* and lead writer for Oprah Winfrey's Super Soul Sunday website

"Anette's story is a page-turner detailing a journey of physical, emotional, and spiritual growth. An engaging and easy-to-read memoir that empowers us all to remember healing is possible."

—Dr. Melanie Joy, PhD, holistic health practitioner

"This is a memoir of sharp contrasts and deep truths: Denmark and America, privilege and loss, health and illness, falling apart and finding one's way back. What shines brightest is Nilsson's hard-won courage and resilience. Her story is both deeply personal and broadly resonant for anyone navigating loss and reinvention."

—Lori Erickson, author of *The Soul of the Family Tree* and *Every Step is Home*

"I've read a lot of memoirs about women who got caught in bad relationships, but few are as honest, sharp, and ultimately uplifting as this one. This is a book about what happens when you stop trying to be perfect and start telling the truth."

—Kay Xander Mellish, author of *How to Live in Denmark* and *Working with Danes*

SOUL-
HAPPY

Published in 2026 by
She Writes Press, an imprint of The Stable Book Group

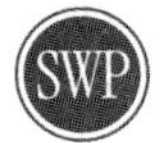

32 Court Street, Suite 2109
Brooklyn, NY 11201
https://shewritespress.com
Library of Congress Control Number: 2025927607
ISBN: 979-8-89636-104-6
eISBN: 979-8-89636-105-3

Interior Designer: Tabitha Lahr

In Chapter 14, the author has included quotes by the following individuals: Philip Dormer Stanhope Chesterfield (1694–1773); George Granville (1666–1735); George Meredith (1828–1909); William Shakespeare (1564–1616); Herbert Samuel (1870–1963). The origins of the poem "Love is many things" and the quote "A wife is a woman who sticks with her husband," from Magnum's notebook, are unknown. Thorough efforts have been made to secure all permissions. Any omissions or corrections will be made in future editions.

Printed in the United States

This book is a memoir. It reflects the author's present recollections of experiences over time. Some names and characteristics have been changed to protect the privacy of individuals, some events have been compressed, and some dialogue has been recreated.

SOUL-HAPPY

A Viking Woman's Long Road Home

ANETTE NILSSON

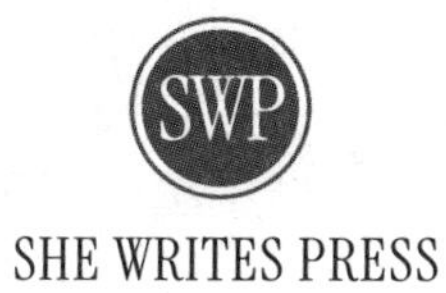

SHE WRITES PRESS

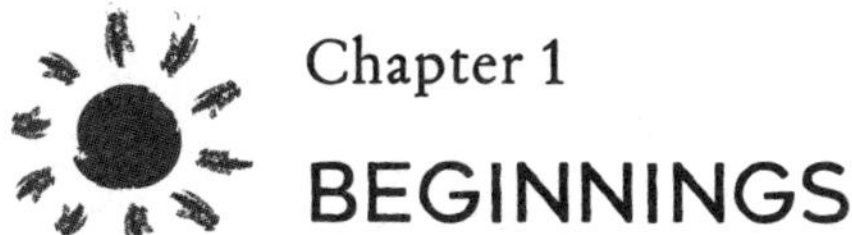

Chapter 1 BEGINNINGS

On a steamy Fourth of July, flags are flying and balloons are dancing in the air along the piers while deep crowds jostle at the railings to join the party. Up and down the Hudson River, people line the water's edge to take in the celebration. Everyone wants to be witness to the biggest tall ship event in history, as well as to the biggest fireworks extravaganza of all time. Today, New York Harbor is the final destination for a grand tour involving thousands of boats—schooners, brigantines, clippers, and three- and four-masters—a congregation of vessels resembling rush hour at Penn Station, which is only blocks away. The crowd's exuberant enjoyment of the festivities and their anticipation of the new millennium fuse into a cacophony that strikes the air like magnificent fireworks.

And here I am, Nette from northern Denmark, not blending into the boisterous, swirling celebration of red, white, and blue but instead sitting quietly below the piers in a gated marina on one of the luxury yachts built for the 1 percent. We are drawing the attention of onlookers almost as much as the tall ships farther out are. Though I am from a place without rivers and extravagance, a place where the seagulls' screech tears the air like a millennial roar, I am sitting on a swanky yacht in the best city in the world, with crowds envying my seat.

"Winners have fucking slips in Chelsea Piers in the biggest goddamn slam ever." The owner's voice shoots across the deck of the *Sun Dancer*, nearly making indentations in the beige leather seat where I am sitting. "It took balls to get this slip on the day when the whole fucking world's watching. I got fuckin' balls. Balls like nobody else! No one can do what I do. Those pock-faced losers up there all wanna be me."

"Yeah, yeah, we know." Liam's hand flies into the cooler and produces two chilled Heinekens. The Igloo cooler and Liam are stock items on the boat. "You got the world by the balls, Cal. Next year, it's a helipad as big as Forbes's. Or bigger. You want another one?"

"Aw, shut up," Cal says, bolting up from the cockpit. The US Coast Guard has banned all regular boat traffic for the remainder of the day, yet he is still toying with the control panel. "I do grunt work producing value for companies, not like those pricks in Silicon Valley—biggest thieves in the world, with their con-dot-com shit that's nothing but air. If you worked as hard as I do instead of wasting your God-given ninety-mile-an-hour pitching arm and scholarships, you'd be playing the Majors right now and making mint. You got nobody to blame but yourself."

My husband is right. About his little brother and about the Fortune 500 companies he has by the balls back in Minneapolis, where we used to live. The tech craze started a few years ago, making the US economy go gangbusters and making us small figures in a time that has boasted inconceivable wealth begotten by the lucky ones, the greedy ones, and the smart ones—a period that has forever changed the world as only a revolution can.

It is a great cover story. But it hasn't always been this way. Before the cover story, before my husband found technology—

or technology found him—we were struggling like many newlyweds.

We met in Denmark, dated between New York and Toronto, and then married in the US and moved to Minnesota, which turned out to be a hub for a tech revolution in supersonic motion. Bill Gates was changing the world then by introducing Windows 95, transforming all transactions. The survival instinct of companies made them spend on IT budgets like sex-starved goons in strip clubs, flinging bills at anything that might produce a bang—big or small, they didn't care. My husband had simply tapped into this, along with his own tech genius.

Boom.

A powerful surge from the bursting, mad river traffic sweeps through the sea wall protecting the marina, rocking the *Sun Dancer*, and jolting hands and legs about on the ivory deck. The unexpected clash pierces something in my own color, beige, and sudden questions erupt.

How did I get stuck in this nightmare life, on this lousy boat, in this grand-slam show of a party I want to escape? How? This was never my dream.

A few moments ago—before the clash from the river, before these madness-driven eruptions, right here on a luxury leather seat under a New York City millennial sky—Calvin's ma, his round, plump Italian ma with her blast of cropped burgundy hair, shocked me into finally feeling something other than the sorry color of beige, a color that's neither hot nor cold, neither a *Yes!* or a *No!* but the dead color of disinterest, of not being anything but soul-unhappy. And not knowing it.

"You didn't know?" she asked. "Calvin got the bump on his nose fixed when he was sixteen. But don't worry, your kids should get your nose. They tend to take after the mother." Maybe it's the scorching July heat or the independence mood that pushed Ma to do what she never before had—slip up and reveal what her son had been hiding from me for years. A nose job.

Who gets a nose job at sixteen? In the seventies? Did they even have plastic surgery then?

In one fell swoop on this hot July 4th day, with the whole world watching from the piers, I feel something that isn't the flat, hollow person that has taken over my body since who knows when. I feel an angry surge of betrayal as if the marine wall has just burst, giving way to the entire mad river inside me—a large body of water gone loose.

How could he? How could he not tell me?

The surge of betrayal blows away the beige cover, and if my in-laws—Ma, Pa, their daughter, Helen, and their youngest son, Liam—weren't on this ivory deck with us, I would dash across to the cockpit and push the man I married overboard. Hoping he'd disappear. Forever.

I don't know the man I married. This is simply one prop too many. Simply one time too many. One of the features I have so admired about him is a lie, a deception he never uncovered—unlike the blue contacts, the seat on the Exchange, the frantic female voice, and the bag of other pretenses that have been brought to light in my company. Perhaps I'd be in Uruguay now, reporting on constitutional turmoil, if he had told me those fine, rounded nostrils and narrow bridge were part of a purchase. But he didn't.

Who is this man?

Ma, Pa, and Helen get up from their seats.

"Did you call for the car?" Helen calls out to her brother. "Ma wants to go home."

There's sudden traffic on the deck now. Liam and his girlfriend are emerging from the stairs to the cabin, and Calvin is heading downstairs. The drill has begun, and I am not the only one who wants to escape.

But I can't. I am stuck. Stuck in this cover story of a successful life, one that seems to have everything and therefore has everything to lose. A mansion on the North Shore of Long Island with six bathrooms, a fancy car and clothes, this yacht and its enviable slip, exploding bank accounts, pipelines bursting with too many projects, and, next up, maybe a private jet lease.

Yet, in the trail left by the mad surge, much like red buoys marking safe water, I suddenly know with the clarity that follows a storm that the anal fissure pain I have been suffering for weeks, bringing me to my knees each time its knifelike pang strikes, refusing to be ignored, is a daily reminder that the weight of the cover story is more than a beige numbness—it is the kind of soul-unhappy that will kill. If not by pushing a husband overboard, then by destroying me from the inside. And I can't last much longer. This situation simply is not survivable. Yet I don't know how to leave. Imagine, a liberated girl from the north who doesn't know how to leave a bad story. How sad.

The Flannerys are debarking the vessel, and I look down at the bundle of velvet joy in my lap. She is the true reason I didn't jump up and push her dad overboard. The beige numbness retracts whenever I look at her, a genuine smile in its place. And more clarity beckons: For her, for her alone, I must find a way. A way out, away, a way back, just some way. A year ago, when she was born, I made her a steadfast promise. Now, I have to find my way so that the weight of the cover story doesn't become hers—a way to be the mama she deserves.

Though I don't yet know it, in this moment, a truth trip is born. A trip to find the power that lies below the cover story that has become mine. A trip that will forever change everything.

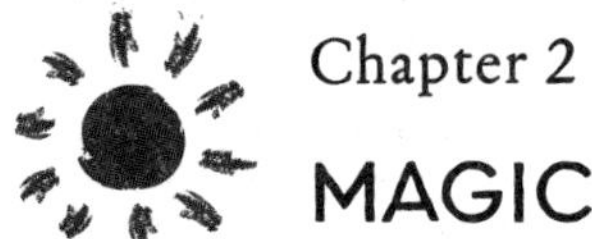

Chapter 2

MAGIC

Some stories have ordinary yet magical beginnings.

It was an afternoon in the mid-seventies in the downstairs of the red-brick house on the corner of Friggsvej. The white shawl of winter softened the almighty darkness that arrived outside the living room windows well before the black-and-white TV set was turned on. Nestled in my spot, snug on the couch next to my mother's father, Morfar, I leaned into the slender arm he wrapped around me.

Mormor, my maternal grandmother, entered the room from the kitchen, carrying a tray full of apple slices she'd cut for us. She joined us before the TV.

Private stations were prohibited in our social democracy; the government wouldn't have anything but one state-funded channel. That was a rule. Sweden, however, was lucky enough to have *two* state channels, and in northern Denmark, antennae could pirate signals from stations across the strait. Sweden was also lucky enough to have a late-afternoon children's show, not like the snowflakes that filled our screen most of the day.

Seconds after Mormor sat down, magic appeared: Emil from Lonneberga emerged on the screen. Generations of children and adults in northern Denmark had learned Swedish by watching the boy with the wooden rifle, tattered blue hat, and indomitable spirit race around the red wooden farm buildings on Katthult, away from the mischief he had gotten into, with a sputtering Father Anton in heavy pursuit, screaming, "*Eeemiiil*" so loud that all of Lonneberga county knew "that Emil" was causing trouble again. Perhaps he had hoisted his little sister, Ida, up on the flagpole so she could see all the way to the neighboring town. Bucolic farm life in early-twentieth-century Sweden brought many opportunities for mischief, and the white-haired, blue-eyed boy always ended up locking himself in the woodshed until Father Anton had cooled down and he himself had carved his latest misdeed into a new wooden figure. Only Alfred, the farmhand, got that the bad-mannered boy was moved by wonder for the world and how it operated. The young boy and the big, quiet farmhand were best friends.

Morfar leaned into me, poking me on the shoulder.

"You," he said in northern dialect just as Emil poured the makings of blood sausage onto Father Anton's head.

We both guffawed. Mormor smiled from her armchair next to us and sipped her chamomile tea. A shawl of warmth wrapped around us, while only the sounds of Katthult and apple munching stayed in the room.

It was magic.

Like Emil, I had white hair, though mine was wild and fluff-like, causing strangers to do double takes as they gawked at the peculiar-looking Danish boy. I hadn't gotten that sweet, angelic girl look. But I was also six years old and insouciant, clearly smitten with life, soul-happy. My blue eyes sparkled because at four, five, and six, imagination takes a young heart where it wishes to go. I roamed the fruit orchard on Friggsvej 6, where a new story unfolded each day—there, nature was the foremost narrator of all. Sparrows nibbling Mormor's breadcrumbs became dragons to conquer among the blaze of orange and yellow marigolds she grew from seed in the spot that signaled summer; the tracks of the porcupine who drank at night from my grandmother's saucer of milk were a curiosity that might lead me to its hidden den. And in the shaded grass below the apple, pear, and plum trees lived a realm of beings, each with a life so amusing that I felt the loud yell of "dinner time" from upstairs was an interference that should be banned.

Some days, I joined the band of fair-haired boys from around the corner, and we roamed as far and wide as our legs and bikes would take us along streets where all the red-brick houses resembled one another. We didn't find trouble, but we found other things. We found an abandoned bus lot, a hermit's smelly backyard, and a way to build a clubhouse from scraps turned up on our roams.

And, sometimes, when mischief crept into me, I found a way to test the universe's complexities all on my own.

"Hey you... Red Tomato!" I yelled at the older boy who lived farther down Friggsvej in what had once been a yellow-brick baker's shop. Red Tomato's flaming hair reminded me of the odious life form stacked next to slivers of cucumbers on my lunch of rye bread. It seemed just right that he got mocked for his bad hair color. Always from a safe distance, though.

This time, however, I got a little too close, and Red Tomato caught up to me on his bike.

"I'll whack you if you call me that one more time!" The pale-skinned, chunky boy lifted clenched knuckles to my face, and I felt his menace of Red.

"I won't—I promise," I mumbled.

Tomato let go of his clenched hands and raced away.

"Hey, you . . . you really look like a big, super-fat red tomato!" I called after him loudly, making sure he heard, before dashing for the safety of my friend Winkie's house.

In a place where the government and neighbors were always in your business, not keeping the neighborly concord was deserving of the big wooden spoon being pulled out in the kitchen upstairs. If Mother Karin heard of my disagreeable behavior toward the boy from Number 33, I would end up getting whacked after all. So I stayed at Winkie's for a while.

Red Tomato later put himself and our little shipyard town in the gusty north on the map by being a pioneer who brought networking and President Clinton to speak at an event in town.

THERE WAS ANOTHER PLACE I used to visit: my very own Katthult. I went whenever Morfar took me in his Opel Kadet to the farm Kirseholt, his second daughter's home.

To get to Kirseholt, we passed through the undulating green terrain that opened up outside Frederik's Harbor—"Frederikshavn" to Danes—our unkingly little town named after a long line of Danish kings. Kirseholt was a magnificent farmstead with whitewashed walls on all buildings, land that stretched to the horizon, and no rules but to explore farming and nature's partnership along with my cousin Tulle, who was two years younger than me. At Kirseholt, the beat of nature ran through every straw in the large, golden haystacks we helped build, and her scent enveloped me as we rolled and rolled and rolled down the meadow against the bright yellow of thousands of dandelions. At Kirseholt, earthy yellowness tickled nostrils, and breath was laughter and soul-happy just was. Everything about nature was real, not fake or covered up. No matter the wind or water, chill or shine, she showed up; every day, I trusted her to be present and to show her unmasked face to me. She was in my DNA, as if she herself had given birth to me, and I had no choice but to love her with all of my being. And I did. *I do.*

Neighbors love rules. Both at Lonneberga and in Frederikshavn and on those afternoons with my grandparents, I guffawed a lot, because again and again Emil defied how a boy from a respectable farm should behave in the world, according to the neighbors. Emil didn't intend to break rules; it simply happened. And perhaps that was how it was for me as well.

I WASN'T YET SIX years old, and I was sitting on the front steps facing the traffic on Friggsvej one early morning.

Mormor belonged to all of us: my family who lived upstairs, my cousins, aunts, uncles, and the brother who was soon to arrive. We all shared her equally. She may have been frugal, having lived through two World Wars, but she squandered on us just the same. She was the subtle strength of our family, an underground mesh that kept us all together, in balance. She was the person we came to for holiday luncheons, Band-Aids for hurt, pranks for parties, and know-how to make everything out of nothing. She was an only child, raised in a well-to-do merchant household of middle-aged adults, and when she directed her table in Friggsvej 6, long rows of descendants and their partners gathered on seats in front of her, her back was erect with the kind of pride that comes when creation is greater than your best dream.

Mormor wasn't always a housewife. In a time when most folks had seldom gone outside Frederikshavn, she had lived and worked in both Copenhagen and Skagen before returning and becoming a local business owner. She was also the first woman in town to get a driver's license and commanded her father's car, known as "Rokken" by townspeople, like a man. She had long been a maiden and had given up on familyhood, her friends already married and mothers, when Aksel showed up. In wartime, with no reason to waste time, in *one, two, three*, a family—a big family—was born.

Indeed, Mormor belonged to all of us. But Morfar—he was a different story. The man with a wavy crop of gold and gray, eyes that winked lapis, and hands that could repair anything was mine alone. And that was undisputed by everyone, even the neighbors.

Each morning, I waited on the front steps for the town bus that he still drove to pass by so I could give him my daily wave. Today was no different.

A couple of bikes with men in blue boiler suits passed by, each carrying a dozen green beer bottles in a plastic bag—a good way to quench your thirst when you worked at the shipyards. Then, the Grouchy Neighbor snuck up on me from around the corner on Halfdansvej, on her way to the grocer's.

I almost missed my chance, but I managed to stick out my tongue in time.

Usually, the Grouchy Neighbor ignored me, but today, she stopped, her face as gray as the sky. "If you do not stop that bad behavior, I am telling your mother," she said. "I do not want to see that bad behavior one more time. Stop it and say you are sorry."

"I'm sorry," I answered, not knowing what that felt like because the Grouchy Neighbor now deserved to see my tongue more than ever.

She yanked her purse and seemed not so grouchy after all as she walked on.

I stayed longer this morning, a patient, white-haired little figure on the concrete steps. When the Grouchy Neighbor returned, she looked at me with a slight smile. Then it happened—just like a glass of milk being knocked over, my tongue popped out again, long enough for her to catch a solid glimpse of it.

That took a little mettle. Though I wasn't yet six, I knew upstairs was sure to hear of my disobedience, and Morfar and

Mormor couldn't save me from the ire of the wooden spoon and Mother Karin's steel-blue eyes. That was a rule.

But the Grouchy Neighbor simply continued on, and she never snarled at me again.

THAT AFTERNOON IN THE warm living room also changed because a *ding-dong* interrupted Emil's mischief on the screen.

A guest at the front door was unusual, as everyone knew to use the back door. I needed to get a first look.

Outside, in the dark chill on the concrete steps, stood a creature slightly older than me. She looked boyish and disheveled; her hair, hands, and clothing were in dirty disarray.

"Where is Dusty?" the urchin asked.

For a moment, I didn't answer. This sure was a guest I hadn't had in mind when I rushed to the door. Dusty was our adorable black poodle, just leaving the puppy stage. How did this impudent urchin know about Dusty?

"He's inside," I finally squeaked.

It got worse. "Is Aksel home?" she asked.

Another affront. How did she know about Morfar? Why was she asking for him? He was my Alfred, and I wouldn't share. If the urchin had her way, she would probably sweep past me to the room that wasn't my room, but was. My bed upstairs was an empty one because I slept most nights downstairs in the narrow bedroom off the hallway, where the bedsheets were ironed and cool and carried Mormor's scent.

The sun fell on me through the small window in the mornings. She wasn't getting in.

"Yes." Another squeak. I felt like hitting her—this audacious rival—in the head with the formal guest door.

After this part, my memory fails me. Perhaps the trauma was too great for me to recall whether the urchin had swept past me in her search for the generous, kind, and caring Morfar, who had struck up a friendship with the neighbor's child, an urchin clearly in need of attention. But later on, I overheard Mother Karin reporting to others that next-door Connie often came to chat with my grandparents and play with Dusty.

I didn't know it then, and wouldn't have cared a hoot anyway at the time, but I'd just had a brush with a celebrity-to-be—the real, made-in-Hollywood, not the Red Tomato local kind. Our little shipyard town, claiming to have the most ferry connections in the world and probably also the most drunken Swedes, was home to actress Connie Nielsen, whose debut was with none other than the smooth, dark, riveting New York Italian Al Pacino, and whose call sheet is still a force to be reckoned with. Or so I've heard. To me, she will always be the urchin who moved into Winkie's house, befriended Morfar against my will, and soon moved out.

At some point, I returned to the warm living room, where Emil was gone for the day. Once more, I was alone with my grandparents. Mormor set the table, and I stayed for slices of rye bread and butter, skipping the homemade liver pate.

Across from me, Morfar heaved a mound of brown sugar onto Mormor's signature rustic bread, a slice for him and a slice for me, that made dessert. When the table was cleared, Mormor returned to her seat with a deck of cards, and we played Five Hundred, a game for young and old, while Morfar occupied his chair by the bay window facing Friggsvej. There in his usual spot, he smoked his pipe, re-read the paper, and fumed a bit over the damned Swedes acting foolish in our streets and the social democratic government, the sure and only things to get his blood boiling.

Mormor and I played on, and soon Morfar was once more soft and mellow. A day was ending, and I headed to my bed in the narrow bedroom. Morfar came to turn off the light because he had a thing for lights, always turning them on and off for me and for generations of my kin. The light has to be just right so you can see your way.

In the dark room, I snuggled against the cool, ironed sheets, and the day left. But the magic stayed.

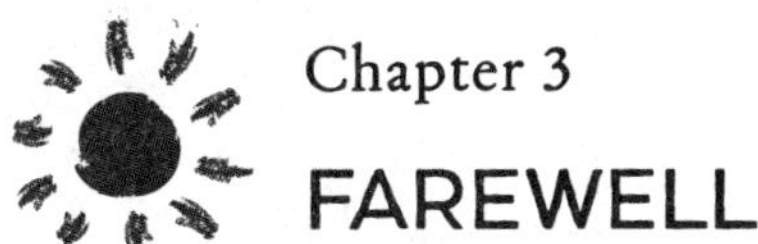

Chapter 3 FAREWELL

In the late 1960s, Canada was a vast land hungry for workers, and it offered cheap airfare loans to industrious Danes who came to make a buck and find adventure. My parents had barely met when my father's contract with the Navy expired.

Nils was twenty-one years old and looking to escape the Danish north. He knew with the unquestioning absoluteness that guides you when you heed the voice of your gut that he wasn't going to end up at the shipyards. That misery was for others, working-class others who didn't think to get away. Besides, the travel bug was in his DNA. His father, Farfar Jarlis, had worked on ships crossing most oceans, and Farfar's own parents had been immigrants from Sweden. His brother Sofus had moved to the Bronx, while another uncle had been a merchant soldier in British-controlled Palestine.

When Nils asked Karin to emigrate with him to Canada a few dates after she, at a local dance, had arranged to bump into the young man in uniform towering over his peers, her gut screamed *no!* to Canada, but *yes!* to Nils. She had to have him, or others would. Before long, they were engaged, and air tickets purchased, and soon after that, they were married and living in an apartment in Park Towers in Mississauga, a suburb of Toronto and home to a colony of other adventure-stricken Danes.

Life in Canada was an adventure, all right. Nils worked for a Danish butcher company, using the skills he'd gained from a long machining apprenticeship on the piers in Frederikshavn, while Karin struggled to use her formal draftsman education. They made pennies that covered rent and payments on a new brown Plymouth Valiant, a sleek workhorse that took them traveling down to the States whenever the butcher was on break. Nils's brother, Jarlis, bragged to his peers on the piers that his older brother had achieved the American dream: a radical car with movie-star looks.

Baby Sallie soon arrived, and she was placed in the work-horse and taken on long road trips down south to discover America.

But one day, the adventure turned bust. Nils entered the apartment after a long shift, perhaps hankering to see his wife cuddling little Sallie and the new baby, Nette—but instead, a frenzied female voice hit him in the entryway.

"I want to go home! I want to go home!"

There was a bang, followed by the jingling sound of shattering glass, and then piercing wails.

Two long strides and Nils was in the living room doorway. "What's going on here?" he demanded.

Shards of glass, former wedding gifts, flew in the air. The usual sureness of his voice—a voice capable of making babies quiver, dogs pee, and Karin fall in love—broke in the air today.

"I want to go home!" Karin's shrieks split the air as she grabbed a frame off the wall and hit it against the plaster until it, too, shattered. "I hate this lousy place . . . I hate it here . . ." Her fashionable blonde pageboy wig flew off as she banged her head against the wall in steady, mad moves.

This wasn't the nineteen-year-old woman from good stock, with calves that made any dress look worthy of Jackie O and a catchy laugh that Nils had fallen for. This wasn't how it was supposed to be. What was happening? His natural brawn, which usually ruled the space around him, was checkmated by Karin's actions. But he had to act. He needed to stop the terrible hysteria seizing his wife. She was hurting herself.

Bang! A big hand landed on Karin's cheek, stunning her into the real world again.

A little while later, Karin's five-year tryst in Canada ended. She took her two daughters back to Denmark. Nils stayed on a while longer to make the buck they'd come for.

This is how it came to be that my family lived upstairs in the house Karin grew up in, and I, a mere ten-month-old, found a way to get out of the crib one night, slide down the steep staircase, and show up in my grandparents' bedroom.

It was a simple choice to pick Morfar's side of the bed. I knew he would fill my bottle, not with water but with the sweet syrup that passed for juice in the seventies. He'd make it so rich and sweet it burnt my young throat. And when I dropped my bottle in the dark, he'd crawl under the bed to rescue it and make everything right.

For the next four years, I made the nightly trip to get my bottle filled, and in doing so, I achieved what my sister or cousins could have done but didn't: I claimed Morfar and made him all mine.

FATHER NILS EVENTUALLY returned from Canada but was soon looking for new adventures. Australia was calling.

This time, Mother Karin heeded the whisper of her gut and said no. She was staying. Father Nils returned to Canada for a while, and then came back and tried settling in a machinist job, not at the shipyards but one town over. He couldn't, however—and he couldn't leave his family for solo adventures in Australia, either.

Then came the lucky break that made everyone get what they wanted: Father Nils was offered a job installing and repairing concrete pipe-producing machines, a job that would take him around the globe 180 days a year and give him the escape and adventure his gut desired. Mother Karin would get to stay in Frederikshavn without needing to find a job. They would even get a sea-green Marina. It was the size of a matchbox car, so tiny we barely fit in it. Yet it was a car, a rare commodity in town, and so earned our family a new level of respect.

Nils got to travel, Karin got to stay, and we got a matchbox car. This development was a happy arrangement, at least for a while.

THE LATE 1970S WERE dark years, set against the Cold War, screaming unemployment, and oil crises that drove the cost of living haywire.

Even so, today was a good day. Father Nils was employed but home for a few days. Mother Karin blared a tune without the accompaniment of the radio in the little kitchen we were soon to leave.

Only I wanted to escape the good day upstairs.

"*There is a suuurpriseee waiiiting fooor youuu*," Mother Karin trumpeted her joy to Sallie, me, and the little brother who had arrived three years earlier—let's call him Penis, since that was seemingly the quality that made him our mother's favorite.

She herded us out the door to meet Father Nils around the corner on Halfdansvej.

"Hello, kiddos." My father's blended scent of shower and Old Spice greeted me with a hug that blew away some of the pouting on my nine-year-old face. He stood in the open front door of Halfdansvej 9, a big hammer and measuring tape in hand, waiting for us.

For the past many months on his visits home, he'd been up earlier than the sun to help get Number 9 into move-in shape. It was an old red-brick, two-family home, and turning it into a domicile akin to a brand-spanking-new single-family house had taken a lot of doing. For months, nay years, crews of craftsmen had appeared to move everything but the four main red-brick walls around to refashion the weathered structure into something that could have been purchased much cheaper.

"Hurry," Mother Karin said, "I can't wait to see your faces." She charged the lacquered custom-built stairs with Sallie, me, and Little Penis trailing behind.

"I've worked hard for this, kiddos. I hope you appreciate it." Father Nils followed us to the second floor, where four bedrooms had popped up. Very small ones, yes, but they would still count as four on the tax sheet.

And there it was. In the middle bedroom that would now replace my room off the hallway stood a surprise so yellow it brightened the room I didn't want to call mine. My grandparents' house had plenty of sleeping spaces, and I couldn't get into my nine-year-old head why we had to leave a home with so many empty beds.

I touched the surprise against the wall—a brand-new desk in bright birch hues and a swivel chair so yellow it matched the sun on its brightest day—and I tried to make friends. But my hands refused. I did love yellow, and that softened the hurt of the surprise that could have pouting turn to tears. But we didn't know tears in my family. That was, you know, a *rule.*

"Isn't it grand? Isn't it wonderful?" Mother Karin's voice exploded through a new paper-thin wall from Sallie's room. Her joy couldn't be mistaken for anything else. "We can't really afford it, but I wanted you to have it. You need desks. Good ones."

In the two other bedrooms stood similar surprises in red and blue. Penis was three years old, too young to appreciate; I was nine years old, too sullen to appreciate. Sallie, now twelve, was perhaps appreciative.

"You like it?" When Father Nils appeared in the doorway of my new place to sleep, I fake-happyed a smile. I disliked when he got a disappointed or stern look in his hazy eyes. He'd worked hard to get us the surprises his wife had asked for, and he just wanted us all to be happy; he said so all the time. He had saved most of his daily dinner allowance from the trips to Poland, East Germany, and Czechoslovakia that took him away from us to spend on this house. He was used to sacrificing, he told us often, because he'd been just six years old when he started delivering papers on the outskirts of town, and his mother had seized every penny he'd earned. She'd had to, or eviction would be next.

My father was the oldest son of a brood of four. Alley Shit, they were called by others almost as poor as they were. That stung. My grandfather, Farfar Jarlis, had unreliable income, even with his schnapps smuggling trade. My grandmother, Farmor, worked four jobs: getting up before the sun, scrubbing floors and washing for others, and using bottles of the potato-based, high-proof alcohol known as schnapps as barter for many goods. Somewhere along the way, she lost the freshness of her oval face, with its features that clung to your memory like the sweet taste of cherry from a bygone summer. So the few extra *øre* earned from the morning efforts of a boy too young to read made a difference.

The paper route eventually turned into an afternoon delivery job on an unwieldy bicycle that stopped my father from playing soccer with other boys in the street. The one afternoon he threw the black iron horse against a hedge and became a nine-year-old boy who forgot about linens wrapped in brown paper on the carrier load of the Long John, Farfar Jarlis's cane came down on him so hard that he never forgot about his job again. The need to be hardworking was literally beaten into young Nils.

So yes, Father Nils got a big smile. And I got one of his warm, wet kisses in return.

BEING NINE YEARS OLD really, really sucked. Life changed after we moved to Halfdansvej 9 and those four tiny bedrooms became ours. The eighties took over, and Yahtzee games and windy walks on the beach with our parents holding hands were discontinued whenever Father Nils's black suitcase showed up in the hallway and stayed for one, even two weeks.

During this time, Sallie became a teenager who beat Father Nils in a race in the Bangsbo woods, where he made us run before dawn when he was home.

Always my opposite—less tall, with brownish hair, hazy eyes, and a jolliness that matched Father Nils's—Sallie also had a big smile, big ears, big feet, and big knockers. She was popular, too, with a gym team, a tennis team, a trumpet team, and a team of boys hankering for her company. They all visited. A lot. Especially the boys. But Sallie didn't listen to her gut and couldn't listen to her dreams, because she wasn't friends with them. Down the line, she listened to Mother Karin, who was afraid her oldest wouldn't get a job amid the crazy unemployment and would become "one of those people." She made Sallie apply for a dental hygienist apprenticeship, which she got easily.

Her fate was polishing instruments and teeth, and that was a fate almost as bad as the shipyards, if you had asked me then.

Mother Karin discovered sewing when a friend invited her to join an evening class on dressmaking. After that, whenever kitchen and cleaning didn't beckon her, she was in the big room in the basement, the needle on her new electric sewing machine roaring across materials that made it a cinch to afford staying stylish, and she heard and saw nothing but the needle until cloth turned to garment.

In the spirit of the eighties, with ABBA and punk setting clothing trends, Mother Karin turned out items that she hoped would make her popular teenage daughter appear chic. She'd once had a volleyball team, a Girl Scout team, and a few other teams of her own, so she knew all about the duty of popularity.

Little Penis was still everyone's darling. He was now a five-year-old who did an afternoon round on the block to three different ladies for cake and card games. He also filled the rooms at Halfdansvej with amiable shouts of Premier League soccer scores and ballgames in the driveway with his teams of friends and a couple of tagalong girls. Indeed, he was just as popular as my sister.

The biggest change, perhaps, happened with Father Nils. He made the Nilsson coffers grow so necessary goods like a better car, a dishwasher, good tennis rackets, and a modern-looking backyard—things his wife knew we needed—could all be purchased. He reminded us often that if he made it to 180 days of travel this year, he would get his taxes back and that he was behind on the days, so he couldn't stay long. In a country where the tax rate was at least 50 percent—even 75 percent, if you were a top earner like Nils—working for a full tax refund was an exceedingly good argument. Indeed, the 180 days of travel were paying off, even if he always seemed behind. He reminded us often how lucky we were to have all the things we had. People in Eastern Europe weren't so fortunate.

Father Nils was also changing because the world outside of him was changing, turning out softer men who could cry. The stern father left—Little Penis never got to feel a smack of the big hand—and his jokes took over full-time. That part was a nice change, and we loved this new version of Father Nils.

ONE FRIDAY EVENING WHEN Father Nils was away, our family acted out what had become a new ritual: Each of us settled on the new couch in the living room just before a favorite American TV show came on. The government had by now relinquished its one-channel monopoly, and we had more stations and shows like *Dynasty* available to us. Mother Karin placed a huge bottle of Coca-Cola on the marble sofa table next to bags of Haribo candy. Sallie's boyfriend, Ulrik, joined us.

"Who are you kissing tonight?" Ulrik taunted me in a twenty-two-year-old voice that felt like the sweet juice that used to burn my throat, making me blush. "You want your first kiss now?"

Ulrik was a mechanic with a mustache and brown eyes that glowed "good time." If I agreed, I knew he would kiss me right there on the sofa with Mother Karin's eyes locked on us and his young girlfriend giggling away. Ulrik always got away with saying things no one else could because he had a magic button that made the female gender go weak and agreeable. Even at our house. But he didn't get away with leaving his green, souped-up Volkswagen outside when he slept over; Mother Karin made him park around the corner because she didn't want the Nielsens across the street to know her fifteen-year-old daughter was having male company at night.

Sallie broke the spell of her boyfriend's delightful taunt. "You look like a donkey with glossy lips. Who are you trying to impress? What's his name?" Her taunt was void of all delight.

You're the ass, and we all know it. I didn't say it, but not because Father Nils had banned all name-calling for years—because Ulrik was sitting next to me, turning his tongue indecently against his red male lips. Instead, I scurried away to wash off my lustrous mistake. I was twelve and didn't hang out with the boy band anymore because our bodies were growing in different directions. Now I was trying to figure out my new direction.

The sparkling new color TV was turned on when I returned; before us lay forty minutes of action-filled drama, no commercials, and the promise of seeing a fatherly look-alike in the lead. Friday evenings were dedicated to *Magnum, P.I.* because Tom Selleck was a close image of our own father. Both were tall, brawny men. They were muscular and broad-shouldered, with every limb big and well-formed, as if shaped by an adoring sculptor. They had handsome features in wide faces, wavy, near-black hair, deep-set, blue eyes, and smiles that stretched from cheek to cheek. Magnum P.I. drove a red Ferrari and lived an unreal, dreamy lifestyle in a guesthouse on an ocean estate in Hawaii, where he came and went according to his desires while investigating mysteries and gallivanting with gorgeous women. Father Nils didn't have dimples, and Mother Karin would never have let him wear a pineapple-print shirt, but otherwise, it was a startling resemblance that fooled us into worshiping Friday evenings, bringing an away husband and a single-mom household closer together—and, for my part, earned Father Nils a new moniker. Henceforth, in my mind, he would always be "Magnum."

"That's grand Hawaii!" Mother Karin announced. She had a thing for ocean and blue water and couldn't ever get enough of it. She made us all go to the West Coast often—our white Volvo with a black roof flying across country roads, for Mother Karin had no doubt about her ability to commandeer a car—because in the spot where the Atlantic Ocean hit the shore of the Danish mainland, the waves were wild and the current would kill, and that was also grand. This setting was the kind of wildness that must be respected; you couldn't refuse the power of that ocean. If you did, the waves and current would swallow you, and you would perish, as German tourists tended to do each summer. Mother Karin could watch the rough beat of the West Coast water for hours.

Although Hawaii-on-the-screen wasn't wild Atlantic but

rather blue Pacific Ocean, its bright, colorful lushness was much like a big bag of Haribo Matador Mix, with its pieces in vivid colors and foreign flavors, and was an instant cheer for Mother Karin—for all of us, really.

IN THE ROOMS AT Halfdansvej 9, it wasn't just Sallie, Magnum, and the world that was changing. I tried to resist, but my body won this battle, and I, too, changed. The scrawny boy-girl with white, kinky floss hair that triggered invectives from friends and strangers left and—overnight, it seemed—a young woman with wavy, white-golden hair, striking black eyebrows, and slanted blue eyes set in a very nice bone structure showed up. Perhaps because this change took place so suddenly, I felt like the good looks weren't really mine but borrowed from somewhere.

I didn't try to be popular, for I loved school. That was a place where you learned about the world and got to write, and that was plenty good. While I and everything around me changed, I made up stories. I made stories up about Canada because I was going there. Since I'd sat on the concrete steps of Friggsvej 6, waiting to give Morfar my daily wave, I had known with an absoluteness so firm and round and bouncy that it was like a ball in my stomach that I would one day leave town, leave for Canada, to find adventure. For fifteen years, I had made up stories about the adventures that lay ahead of me in the place where I was born.

It may not seem like a big deal to plan to go to Canada after high school. But in Denmark in the early eighties, it was. The world was still segregated into distinct continents, and the link of communication between them was an expensive commodity, a rarity that had to be saved up for or meted out in calculated minutes from or to a father in Czechoslovakia and other lands. The world consisted of foreign places and faraway, unknown life that you couldn't access in seconds with a handheld device.

Somewhere in this huge, removed world sat little *Danmark*, a socialist country unto its own. And living in a small socialist country required conformity. *Conform or be ostracized* was a rule we all knew. For me, dumb rules and conformity felt like stylish clothes with too-tight seams that I didn't want to wear, so leaving was something I was skip-happy longing for.

Teachers and others who paid attention had always known I was going places. In the north, however, you couldn't go places, and striving was certainly not a socialist value, so when you had the kind of dreams, drive, and decidedness that teachers and others recognized because it didn't come around often, there was no choice but to go out into the world to make space for it. That was what I planned to do.

While I was waiting to go, the reveries in my Canadian stories spanned the horizon of all the dreams a woolly-headed, highly imaginative girl from a gusty shipyard town could conjure up. The early stories involved a herd of horses, helicopters, and a ranch in western Canada by the Rockies. In the Magnum years, when my father traveled a lot to Czechoslovakia and considered smuggling a violin out through the Iron Curtain like a 007 father, they turned to international spy business. The last set featured a modern-day Tarzan I was destined to meet on the streets in Toronto.

Our family had made a one-of-a-kind trip to Canada the summer when I was thirteen, so I knew very well the down-town corner where we were going to meet. Tarzan would be so captivated by my inner and outer beauty that we'd hold hands and go to the jungle, where I, too, would learn Animal-Speak.

Interwoven with all these stories was one thread, a true affection that could not be hemmed in no matter my age or changes, and that was my yellow typewriter, an electric version of the mechanical one Magnum beat away at when he was home, upon which I fashioned stories that stirred people to see something new. I was an author, a writer, and finally, a journalist working for *The New York Times*, traveling to unknown corners of the world to report on crises that otherwise would be ignored.

But before I went, a real-life Tarzan showed up and captured my heart for a while.

IT WAS MAY, BIRDS were nesting, I was nearly seventeen, and the wavy white-golden hair had descended on me. I'd had one Carlsberg at the annual public tent party by the stadium, and the DJ played Rick Astley's "Wanna Dance with Me?" when a pair of big, sculpted hands heaved me up on one of the wooden benches where townsfolk of all ages drank from green bottles ad libitum.

I didn't want to dance, because who was this . . . *wait!*

Seconds later, I did want to dance. In fact, Rune and I danced the rest of the night, on and off the benches, because he enjoyed the disco beat as much as I did.

I couldn't miss that Rune resembled the Tarzan of my stories. He had a perfect body—long, lean, and muscular from years of soccer practice, while nature had endowed him with perfect V-shaped proportions of shoulders, butt, and everything else. He was perfect brawn, like Tarzan. And that evening I learned how well-trained pecs could make me quiver and raise my heartbeat to dangerous levels. Rune was simply a gorgeous twenty-one-year-old hunk of young man who, for inexplicable reasons, had trekked to Frederikshavn from Randers, a city more than an hour away, for our annual party.

I got my first real kiss, and later much, much more, from that dark-haired, green-eyed Tarzan look-alike who wore a military uniform on working days.

Within a few weeks, it was clear to us both that this was love. And lust. I never for a moment doubted that Rune adored me without measure. And I him. We always made things right when they went wrong between us, as they often did.

But Rune couldn't keep me. The ball in my gut was too bouncy, the dreams too long, and the rules too many.

Still, he tried.

"Wanna get married?" he asked a short while after I had turned eighteen, and his contract with the military was up but had been replaced with a polishing-weapons contract. He, too, was a machinist.

For half a tick, I entertained his proposal. Below my breastbone was a spot that cried, even begged, to stay, because not being wrapped in Rune's strong, beautiful body that loved me so and never asked me to change a thing wanted it all to go on. His brawn against mine, forever. But the rest of me screamed, *No!* Rune never wanted to leave Randers, and he drank a lot of Tuborg, a favorite national beer. In fact, *we* drank a lot of Tuborg, and we partied with his teams of guy friends every weekend. That was fun for now, but for Rune it was forever. This was his way.

The summer before my last high school year, I visited family friends outside Toronto, a trip I'd saved up for and made happen on my own. While I was away, Rune claimed he was bereaved and took a bank loan to go to a popular beach town with enough dough to drink ad nauseum for his two weeks of vacation. That kind of money could have sponsored a trip to a remote land, but Rune liked caravan camping inside Danish borders, preferably in the north, with coolers of Tuborg.

That was it. First Love didn't stand a chance, and I left. The reason in my gut had to be given a place to live.

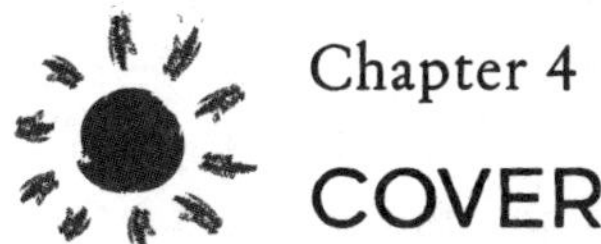

Chapter 4
COVER

"Hey, girls!" I threw my book bag on the floor and slipped into a seat at the bar next to two fair-haired maidens drinking from red plastic cups. "Did you get any cock recently?"

I was twenty, and life had changed once again. I was living my Canadian stories smack in the middle of downtown Toronto. The urban sprawl of the city had become home.

A cough seized Dahlia, beer clogging her throat. Soon, a grin overwhelmed her Danish face—pretty red cheeks, blue eyes, and all. She turned to the other girl and gave her a high five. "She's cool!"

Camilla's cheers lightened her face, too, as she said, "Shut up. We thought you were a schoolgirl. Have some Molson." She pushed a red plastic cup toward me and swayed her body to the music from the man-size speaker across from us. "It's a good place you picked out."

"Yeah, we oughtta be able to find some Canadian dick in here." Dahlia swung around to face a medley of ripped jeans, heavy sweaters, baseball caps, trails of cups, and rave lights joined in a tumult of speed drinking, dancing, and pool-playing. We were in frat territory, in a place with absolutely no presence of rules, and U2's "Mysterious Ways" was playing. It was, after all, 1991.

Madison House—a labyrinth of countless rooms, patios, staircases, and student beds—was a Victorian mansion turned bar on the University of Toronto campus. I was a student in my second year of studies. And I'd seen just about everything—that is, anything involving beer, sex, and young people—happen here.

I'd made friends in my new home—a couple of students in their junior year, some other Canadians, and now also Dahlia and Camilla, who were trying out Canada by working illegally as au pairs—since making my escape three years earlier. It'd been a no-brainer for me to move to my birth town. While I was finishing up high school, a call to the embassy confirmed that a leak in Danish law conferred me rights to a Canadian passport. Following that, I'd placed an ad in the *Toronto Star* newspaper, and soon afterward had received a stack of letters with nanny job offerings.

During my first three months in Toronto, I worked for a South African expat family while taking classes at Ryerson, a technical institute that accepted late applications. A while later, I had upgraded to the University of Toronto, where I then pursued a dual-degree bachelor—prep work for a master's in journalism. I squeezed time in between two jobs and school for nights out like this one.

"How's university?" Camilla's interest was genuine. One day, she might enroll in something.

I sipped from the red cup and then let out what I'd been keeping to myself: "It's absolutely the hardest thing I've ever done. Everything's different, and you never know what to expect when you walk into a classroom. Even the ink cartridges on the school typewriters are different, and you have to bring a cartridge yourself. Plus, writing English at uni level—that's a whole other world from what the DK school system teaches. It's real hard."

I paused again, enjoying the track change. George Michael's

"Freedom" moved through the room, sounding almost as great as when I'd seen him live in Gothenburg, across the strait from Frederikshavn. "Still, it's hands down the best thing I've ever done. I love it here! I wouldn't change a thing."

"Shut up, you two. Let's party for real. I wanna score someone." Dahlia slurred, though her smile and party zest were still as catchy as George Michael's tune.

And we did. We danced, and we scored.

Alongside Camilla and Dahlia, I learned what it was like to fuck someone you'd just met, using the fuck-as-you-go method that was the way of my peers back home.

In Denmark, fucking was cool. Fucking was power. Our country was a birthplace of sexual freedoms, and at home, young women acted just like men since women and porn were free now. In high school there had been plenty of cute local boys, but none had seemed worthy of a piece of my essence. Only Tarzan could have all of me, all that was too sacred to be let out in public.

But now, I, too, started acting from the Danish promiscuity wound, confusing promiscuous sex with self-power and love. No one ever told me that empowerment isn't achieved by doing reflexively what others do. But for a while, my adventures with my girlfriends had me convinced that fake empowerment was its own thrill and tale.

MAYBE ALL TEENAGERS have a moment when they are at an abrupt crossroads, and their direction is either continued or abandoned because life is changing, and they can no longer touch the place inside where truth resides.

My crossroads moment happened not long after I, at sixteen, started Gymnasium, the academic high school that supported an ambition for going places. I was surrounded by a world of unfamiliar kids, all with some sort of intention other than an apprenticeship or a dead-end job. I was very lucky, because I got to go there. I got to do what young Nils hadn't gotten to do. This was another way in which my father had sacrificed, and it was one tough to understand, let alone accept.

Young Nils, too, loved school. He loved it so much that he'd skipped a grade. And was possibly going to skip another grade after that—well, he did. He skipped out of seventh grade altogether, and the option to enter Realskolen, the Gymnasium equivalent at the time, was never his.

Farmor surprised him one day at dinner with an order to show up at Bjerg's the next morning rather than go to school. She'd negotiated an apprenticeship for him because, once again, she needed his earnings. Better earnings, mind you. Her husband had just died.

If Farfar had beaten the lung trouble that came from shoveling coals on steamers, he would have overruled Nancy—or Nanghsi, as she was known. He would have ruled that Nils go to Realskolen, where his abilities belonged, and not at the piers, where he ended up. Farfar Jarlis was a man of principle, not Nanghsi-like pragmatism. He brought home books from travels and had his daughter take ballroom dance classes and Nils music lessons, though the coffers were barren. Perhaps his mixed roots were what made him so.

His father was Lars Nilsson, a handsome hulk of a Swedish day laborer who fell deeply in love with an aristocrat, the fair Anna Emilia. Her family disowned her, so the young couple eloped across the strait to Denmark, where foreigners, even if of Viking stock, were treated worse than stray dogs in the late 1800s. Lars—my great-grandfather—became a stonemason, an occupation reserved for the poorest, most desperate, and toughest, yet still managed to raise six children with his wife. And a piece of Lars and Anna Emilia lodged in Farfar Jarlis. He, too, was forced into blue-collar existence, but part of him had been shown the way of the aristocrat. Love of learning and culture was a spark in him, and he would have defied societal rules and Nanghsi and have his son enter the place where he belonged, among books and erudition.

Farfar didn't make it, and neither did young Nils. But now I got to be here.

I had to give it my all, for myself and for the memory of those before me who couldn't. Each day that I skipped up the concrete steps to the front door, I was driven to be among the best in each class. That was a lot of drive because there were plenty of other studious kids. Worse still, many of these studious kids were cool. The kind of cool that came with almost being an adult who could drink and party hard and do whatever because a legal right was a legal right, and because we were choosing to leave ordinary town life behind. No fear of a nuclear war or a dead Amazon could quell the youthful optimism that the future was ours to mold. So, when you were sixteen and had just started Gymnasium in Frederikshavn in 1986, you owned life. And you let it be known.

Red-haired Mette, with her big freckles that left her neither pretty nor likable and yet somehow very cool, had me at my crossroads moment.

At break time, a handful of classmates were gathered around a table while waiting for German class to begin. Only three guys had made it into our class, and none of them were around today.

"I bonked Hans last night . . . *ooh la la*, it was great!" There was no mistaking Mette's indulgence in last night's event. Her freckled face was fluorescent with pleasure, and her voice boasted experience.

"Oh yeah—he's got a big dick. I did him last week," Signe, who knew the German textbook best of anyone, chimed in. "Did anyone do the assigned conjugations?"

Gitte, with her mint cowboy boots and doe eyes, checked her homework against Signe's as she added to the table talk. "I'm gonna ride Morten next time he's at Unik Disco. Who's coming Saturday? Let's get plastered and go get dick."

"Girls," a deep male voice interrupted, "let's focus on our conjugations and not on this weekend's screwing party, even if it sounds alluring." Teacher Johannes had shown up. "Signe, conjugate verbs from yesterday, *bitte*."

During Signe's perfect conjugations of a long list of unusual German verbs, it dawned on me that everyone but me was having sex, and I suddenly realized: I was many things, but I was not cool. And that had to change.

It never occurred to me to ask whether others were at their crossroads moment, too. For once, I didn't beg a question. Outrunning the joint forces of conformity and promiscuity was tough when you were sixteen and wanted to succeed at Gymnasium.

This was how my story twisted, and my cover story started.

IN MY TEENS, COOL simply happened to be fucking someone you'd just met. Danish toddlerhood began with meeting hardcore porn in open view on counters and shelves at the corner store where Mom fetched milk. Our keen notion of sexual freedom shaped us all like a brook running through a landscape, moving and molding the soil along its path. Our country's love of sexual freedom was nearly impossible to outrun. Even in the Danish Seamen's Church in the northern outskirts of Toronto, where I was baptized and where I went one wintry evening after receiving an invitation for a meet-and-greet with other young Danes, it showed up. Here, I met Dahlia and Camilla for the first time, and the new pastor was perhaps a little nervous being in a room full of females just a few years younger than himself.

Psalms or prayers weren't on the table that night. But Tuborg was. The pastor opened the meet-and-greet with a green bottle and a simple question: "So, have any of you had sex recently?"

Choked silence; the question rang amongst the crowd of young women far from home with unsettling effect.

No one answered the pastor's question, and maybe that was why I asked it again at Madison that night with Camilla and Dahlia.

The brook kept running through us, almost like a rule. Even in Toronto.

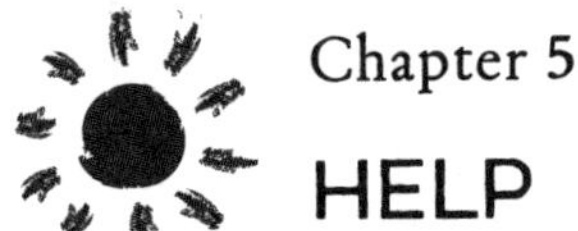

Chapter 5
HELP

A good decade after my crossroads moment, I—we—live on Long Island's North Shore in a mansion with a circular driveway in a town that boasts being the sixth-wealthiest zip code in the US, with a top-notch school system and a marina to match. The Long Island marina is a short boat ride from Chelsea Piers Marina in Manhattan, where we dock whenever my husband's in town. His business is in Minneapolis. The tech revolution is still hanging on, although I cashed out and turned mama more than a year ago.

The searing pain from last summer—an anal fissure caused by a botched colonoscopy—hangs on still and has acquired a few companions: a village of hemorrhoids, stomach cramps, and inescapable diarrhea. Each is agonizing in its own way. But the pain is dwarfed by my own shadow, which I met just a few days ago. I was carrying bags of Whole Foods groceries from our black Jeep through the oak door of our home, feeling as heavy as the brown bags myself, when a thought jumped out at me as if it were a ripe apple leaping out of the bag and rolling on the floor, waiting to be captured: *I don't recognize myself!* If I met myself at a party, I'd think, *Help, let me find someone who's alive.*

That's me now. The happy-go-lucky girl who enthralled an American into a marriage proposal and who was gung-ho about life is gone. In her place is a figure of beige. A person whom I no longer recognize.

I am still stuck. Nothing has changed since the millennial celebration almost a year ago. I have not found a way—in, out, anywhere, let alone away. My strong, tall frame and Viking blood can no longer fend off the physical toll of being soul-unhappy.

The grocery bags are a challenge for reasons other than the weight of beige: I've turned feeble to the point that I can no longer carry the bundle of velvet joy, even when she pleads for a ride in my embrace. If that doesn't kill me, the guilt will. The little toddler girl who greets me each morning with a hug and a sunburst laugh was promised much more than a mansion in a top-notch school district. That I still recognize. For months, I've been trying to make good on that promise and get unstuck. I now can tell the difference between loving and loathing, and there's a whole lot of loathing for my husband mixed in with my beige.

I've acquired a babysitter, I've been to doctors, and I've been to alternative medicine practitioners, all of whom have given me their views and things in little bottles. None of them have done a darn thing, because all my Viking frame wants to do is lie down and rest after a trip to the grocery store just down the road—and I do.

That's not improvement, so medicine, old or new, has no solution for me.

Somewhere in the months since the millennial celebration, another thought has also struck and stuck. Several times a day, anal pain brings me to the edge of fainting unless I dash for the master bathtub, fill it with the hottest water possible, and soak in the heat, joining with a soft mist of lavender essential oil, until the unbearable turns bearable. The baths have forced a space where insight unfolds, spreading inside of me until the insight is all I know and trust. I trust now that becoming unstuck is something other than physical. Something in my soul is not right. And that makes the anal pain and its companion ailments not physical but spiritual at their core. They are expressions of soul-unhappiness. That is why medicine is not a solution. Because it cannot fix my soul. That's on me, entirely on me.

If the lavender mist alone isn't telling me this, my sister is.

Sallie joined the dream of a gym team member and went to California to be a nanny just before I escaped to Canada. Her fabulous year in Southern California led to a marriage to an heir to a Midwestern concrete dynasty, young Dean. After their marriage, Sallie moved from Cali to upstate Michigan, a place where people own snowmobile suits, not surfboards. Soon, a baby boy was born, along with great bowel ailments. Homesickness struck, a divorce followed, and Sallie's tryst in the US ended when she and toddler Cody moved to live with Mother Karin and Little Penis. By the mid-nineties, another shift had taken place in Sallie and the world around her; new-fashioned ideas of otherworld wisdom became accessible way up north, and Sallie gave up fashion and found numerology and personal development.

I don't know how much she transformed at the core during this time, but she did begin wearing loose clothing and ergonomically shaped footwear, like other social workers, and try parachute jumping—which was somehow, she said, intricately tied to her self-worth. Her transformation was aborted around the time she ended up with a waiter and had another son by him. But before that happened, she shared sufficient ideas to inspire me to search for answers to my unhappiness in a place where medical degrees won't go.

Which is also why I, on this bright May day in 2001, have given in to seeing the name on the paper that my babysitter,

Kathleen, handed me a couple of weeks ago. Desperation, Sallie's sharing, and the lavender mist make me seek out Lynn Leclere, who has an office one town over on Main Street, close to the clock tower.

Lynn Leclere is a woman who changes people. That's what Kathleen says. Kathleen's someone I trust when it comes to changing because she changed herself from being a drug and alcohol addict who would do anything to score anything to being squeaky clean and loving kids as much as she used to love a high. She's kept this sober lifestyle up for more than twenty years, so I trust her when it comes to changing what isn't right in your soul.

Today, the gut knot is bigger than normal, because Lynn is a medium. That means souls not-in-this-world speak to her. They tell her things. That's outright something Mother Karin and I have shunned for years. I'm pretty sure Mother Karin used to hear souls whisper, and that was reason enough to shun them, the way she shuns other scary memories that will own a piece of you if you let them in.

Yet here I am at Lynn's door, willing to believe, willing to open up to whatever is. I don't know what to expect, but I do hope for change, the kind that will heal an unbearable anal pain and get me unstuck. The kind that will help me find the real me and bring her back.

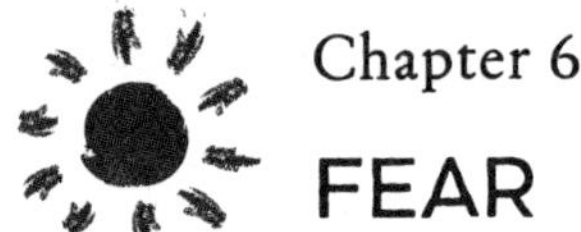

Chapter 6
FEAR

Being a practitioner of the supernatural in 2001 is just short of modern leprosy. A few people find you fascinating, but most wish to dodge someone who claims dead people speak through her. Maybe that's why Lynn was willing to take a test from an accredited institution that uses science to score so-called mediums' ability to channel verifiable information. She scored so high that it shattered all precedent and earned her an immediate phone call from the science department because they had never before encountered someone like her. But these details I don't yet know.

I enter the basement door and find myself in a dark room lit up by strings of white Christmas lights. My heart speeds up then stops, speeds up, and—

"Hi," a voice interrupts my heart's stop-and-sprint mode. "I'm Lynn. How do you pronounce your name?"

In a flash, everything inside gears down and relaxes into nature's rhythm. I have nothing to worry about. In front of me is the warmest glow of a smile I've ever come upon. A smile I trust even before I get to answer her. I follow this winsome woman—she is a decade older than me, with ample curves—into a narrow treatment room, where I lie down on a massage table.

Then Lynn changes my life.

"You pray a lot." Her eyes are closed, and she no longer smiles.

"*Hmm.*" Danes don't admit to praying. Myself included. It's outright embarrassing in a country where the church is an item added to your tax burden and only attended for the trinity of baptism, wedding, and funeral. And perhaps Christmas. All that still sticks with me, even if I did have the velvet bundle baptized in St. Mary's Basilica in Minneapolis, giving her the option of being a Catholic later on. Lutherans don't care which church you call yours. Neither do I.

Still with eyes shut and a voice that wanders to and from someplace else, Lynn states, "You're a good person, very sweet, and your heart's pure."

"Yeah, say that to my husband and see what he says," I intend to say. But I can't. Because I am choking on an avalanche of wetness that comes out of a deep nowhere as if Lynn has pressed a hidden spring in my body and released so many tears that they have flooded my throat.

Though I come from a place that doesn't know tears, the feeling is not unpleasant. In the dark room, Lynn makes everything right. Love comes in many versions, and Lynn's presence makes it known that she's someone who keeps her version for the person on the massage bed. It feels so right that I let the avalanche go.

Lynn snaps me into the dark room again. "Your grandfather is here. You're the apple of his eye. You brought him so much joy. He loves you so! He wants to make sure you understand."

In the dark room, I am given the eyes of my Morfar, and the only picture that exists of young Nette in a dress flashes before me: I am six years old, standing on the concrete steps by the back door in a yellow sundress with blue polka dots. I see how this little girl with white, untamable hair, a good sprinkle of mischief in her eyes, a smile that pleads to play with life, and the faithfulness of four legs trailing you has made herself the apple of her grandfather's beautiful eyes. Her innocence lights up his old age, and the two are a pair with a tie that started with a bottle but grew into something so wide and profound I know only one thing to compare it to: motherhood. As a parent now myself, I see that, indeed, Morfar was right. I did bring him so much joy.

Next to me, Lynn pauses while some other place downloads more imagery into her. Even if I want to think this woman is a hoax and she simply knows how to sweet-talk someone with unbearable pain into believing in her abilities while paying a fine dollar for her services, I can *only* believe her. My Morfar is dead. He died the worst year of my life, back in 1994, when I escaped Denmark again and moved back to the US with my just-married-to husband. But he isn't really gone because it *is* Morfar Lynn is receiving from—it cannot but be so—because she says, "He wants you to take more driving lessons. He's showing you racing down the streets in town, not obeying very many traffic rules." Then she buckles because Morfar's guffaw is so irresistible that it makes an implausible leap through to the physical world and has Lynn in stitches.

I know the guffaw, and I get the joke. No one else knows about it. Like so many other things, it was ours alone.

Morfar made his own escape off a farmstead so small it barely was a farmstead. His passport was getting a rare driver's license, which provided him a ticket to better employment than farming on land too meager to cultivate anything but economic hardship. Young Aksel toured Denmark on his motorcycle, getting into mishaps with his two-wheeled vehicle and women, but by the time he settled down with the Brewer's Ella, his unruly driving habits had settled along with him.

When I turned eighteen, I took driving lessons and passed a driver's test—an extremely stringent one, because rules are many when it comes to Danish driving. Morfar was by then retired and the owner of a sand-colored Opel Kadet, a small sedan he nursed no better or worse than a mother nursing her newborn.

In our family, we knew sharing—except Morfar didn't when it came to his Opel Kadet. The vehicle took him, Mormor, and often me to visit their two other children, on trips to the woods, and to the cemetery, but he never allowed me to touch the wheel. Until one afternoon, Morfar suddenly knew how to share. He asked me to drive his Opel Kadet with him, rather remarkably, occupying the passenger's seat. Also remarkable was all he overcame to ask me to commandeer the Kadet out of town and onto country roads, where we met the undulating green of Frederikshavn's surrounding terrain.

For several more afternoons, Morfar took the passenger's seat while I cautiously guided the sand-colored Kadet along those country roads, all without ever going above the speed limit and always stopping well in time before any light turned from green, my foot a tender touch on the brake.

One afternoon, instead of taking his seat, Morfar poked me on the shoulder.

"You," he said in his northern dialect and guffawed. "Here are the keys. Take the car whenever you want." A pause, because Morfar was after all from the north, where silence is the longest part of conversation. "Nette, you are a good driver."

With the other set of Morfar's car keys in my hand, I realized I'd just passed a second driver's test, one even more stringent and important than the official kind. No one else got what I got. Not Mormor, not Mother Karin, not her siblings, and none of my cousins ever got a chance to show Morfar what a good driver they were. More bikes still swept past the house on Friggsvej than cars, and none of my peers had keys to wheels. Now I did. All my gratitude was fitted into a "*Tak*, Morfar," which in a different family would have been issued in a hug so long that the seagulls turned still.

In the treatment room, I recall that I never did use Morfar's car keys because suddenly I had another set: Magnum and Mother Karin had upgraded to a new Toyota but didn't have the heart to let go of the aging Volvo that had carried us on trips to corners of Denmark that Magnum had wanted us to see and on trips to Skiveren when Mother Karin needed to feel the wild beat of the ocean. They handed the keys over to me.

The Volvo, dubbed White Rocket, still had spark left. I was eighteen, and afternoon upon afternoon, I zipped out of town with my friend Lotte to go to the stables in the middle of the undulating green where she had her horse, and I leased a former racehorse, and we made gaiety like two BFFs do in the last months of high school. The White Rocket flew across country roads, and I forgot all about a tender touch on the brake.

After a few afternoons of this hard driving, the Rocket's spark was challenged. By the time we reached the town sign for Frederikshavn on our return trip, it huffed and puffed like a real racehorse just turned champion. Lotte and I ignored the unsettling white escaping from the hood.

I never had to ask. Morfar was waiting by the curb for the Rocket to arrive that afternoon, lapis glinting at me as I got out, and he lifted the hood to release billows of smoke.

"Let's see what I can do," he said. "It might take a while."

I went to do homework, and later, when I skipped over to Friggsvej 6 for my evening visit, Morfar's clever, gnarled hands handed me the keys. My Rocket was as good as new again.

Until the afternoon that it wasn't. That day, the Rocket began huffing and puffing long before reaching the town sign, and smoke, impossible to ignore, escaped from the hood. As I turned onto Halfdansvej, I forgot all about Morfar by the curb. I forced the gas pedal way down, making the White Rocket bounce into its spot, and ended with a hard foot on the brake—rather inelegant driving.

Morfar responded as only my Morfar would: "You." Pause. "I think you need a few more driving lessons." Then he guffawed, his entire body shaking with merriment and his unbound laugh taking me along. He remembered all about being young and having your first wheels and making them fly like a champion racehorse.

The White Rocket never recovered, and I never got more driving lessons because soon after, I graduated and went to Canada.

But before I moved to Toronto in July of 1988, Morfar showed me who he was, should I have ever had any doubts. I entered the living room one afternoon when he was sitting by the window, embers in his pipe and Mormor's tray with coffee before him, the paper already read and folded. Mormor was in the garden, and I sat down at the mahogany table, host to years of dinners and card games. Just now, the glee in me, the glee of going, was gone. I found myself struggling with my vocal cords. Hours before, when I'd told Mother Karin of my permanent leave plan, she'd reacted not unlike the Atlantic Ocean when it thrashed the western shore with wild beats. My own heart still hadn't recovered nature's rhythm.

I looked at Morfar. His long hands had become ever more gnarled, and all gold had by now left his hair. He was spending more time in the seat by the bay window, and somewhere between us was an ache so deep and wide it must be shunned—because who would go to the woods with him or hold the screwdriver while his unsteady hands attempted a repair? Who would run through political news, even if his rants were fewer since both the drunken Swedes and social democratic government were no longer present? Who would check in on him and Mormor in the evenings? Others would, but not like I would.

There was no pause in Morfar today. He looked straight at me when he said, "Nette, I completely understand. There's nothing here for you in this town, but there's a whole world waiting for you outside. Of course, you must go."

I think it broke his heart to speak those words.

I know they broke mine.

Which is also why I trust what comes next. Morfar may be speaking through a woman I just met in a narrow treatment room on Long Island, but I trust him like no other. He's on my team, forever on my team.

"He says you are unhappy. And your physical woes are emotional." Lynn pauses like someone in the north would, and then continues, "He says over and over that you must get away. If you stay, it will be the end of you. Understand?"

Lynn isn't expecting an answer. She presses on.

"He says you're living in constant fear. That's why you're not getting a divorce. You're letting fear drive your life. It has you in prison—'a convenient prison,' your grandfather says."

In an instant, something I have been ignoring, covering, surfaces. I *am* afraid. I am gripped by fear—fear of leaving, fear of standing on my own in a foreign country with a toddler and no important career. Most of all, I fear having no excuses for not following my dreams, or perhaps I fear following my dreams and failing. Because I was supposed to be going places. The boat and the mansion are places, of course. Neither one was where I intended or wanted to go, but both were convenient. The fear in me is something that no longer will be ignored, however, and I recognize it as one would recognize goose bumps, an itchy scalp, or an avalanche of tears. Except it isn't innocuous; it's insidious. Morfar is right. Fear has me stuck.

"Your pain will increase if you stay, your grandfather says," Lynn speaks clearly. "If you brave a divorce, you will heal. Can you free yourself from fear?"

"I completely get it," I sob into the room's darkness. "Oh, do I get it."

Morfar's telling me to get a divorce. He's telling me truth, and he's telling me much more. He's telling me *dare*, because he knows me best. He knows me from when fear wasn't swallowing my nature. He knows the Nette who can't resist a dare, be it out of fearlessness, recklessness, or inexperience. He knows the Nette who can't help but try to prove what someone questions she can do. He knows I am still the little girl who disproved Winkie and made the dentist's hand bleed to get out of the chair and tooth checking. And he knows how to help her find a way to move fear out of the driver's seat. By daring me. Daring me to have the courage to fight fear in the name of the freedom that always has been an impulse, like another heartbeat, for me.

Sometimes, a dare is how you get to truth.

In the room's silence, imagery falls into me from a time when fear wasn't my nature. *Is this when freedom turned to fear?*

The date picker for this memory shows July 31, 1991, nearly a decade ago to the day. It was the break of dawn. I was skipping naked in the lazy waves of the Baltic Sea on the eastern coast, where wildness never reached. The summer-warm water around my shins broke through the haze in my brain. A naked male body stood next to me, hands thrown into the still air. "I am free . . . I am free . . . I am free." Dawn and yells crossed while the ocean caressed us both. The two cool cover stories that had met a couple of hours earlier over ample shots of tequila at Downtown, a discotheque in the city of Aarhus, were dumped along with scattered clothing in the sand behind us. In this terrific moment, a Viking and a North American skipped and stood together in their own skin, feeling altogether free, and with the ancient ocean as witness. The male body greeted the rising sun with another howl—"I am a fucking Viking!"

I was stupid, I was naive, I was doomed, I was all of the above as I bent down and interrupted the naked male body in his sun salutation.

"Look how tiny it's become," I said, my finger pointed at his manhood. I found it outright curious how the male skin responded when bared against daybreak. No Viking howl could make a North American penis stop nature's reaction. What a funny change.

As if stung by a brute foreign object, the American leaped out of the water and sped across the sand to reach his clothing. The tone of his shouts had changed, all freedom gone. "What the fuck are you doing?" His back was against me as he hurried to put on his white shorts, but I heard him without effort. "What a bitch! What a fucking bitch!"

Just before the tequila haze set in again, I do recall feeling betrayed by my curiosity. It killed the moment with a naked male body full of dawn and ocean next to me, which was never my intent. I couldn't tell the American that, however, because I suddenly found myself in the sand, on my back. The American was on me, in me. Maybe I was enjoying it for a moment, I don't know. The tequila haze was dense and only let in brief bursts of recollection in the treatment room. Here is one:

"I'm not a freakin' doll," I scream out. "I'm not a freakin' Raggedy Ann." A spiky rush growing in the sand cut my back, insulting my skin.

The next burst shows me gathering my jeans and boots somewhere around us.

Stinging, fury, and tears blend in another snapshot.

This sort of sex wasn't my thing. Even through the tequila haze, I knew this.

My anger was short-lived, it seemed, although the American's wasn't. Now fully clothed and getting into the black BMW that was taking him through Europe on business, he was still distorting the fresh morning air with rants of, "What a real fucking bitch!"

A burst of distress appeared. I didn't want to be left behind on a beach in a city I didn't know with no way of getting back to Dahlia's studio apartment, where I'd arrived only yesterday. This made no sense, considering that I had happily moved to a foreign continent without any map but a dream. But it was so.

"You're not fucking getting in," the American yelled shrilly when I attempted to open the door.

"You're going to leave me here? I don't remember where my friend lives." Ten years later, in the treatment room, this recollection is making my toes twitch and curl. Because now I know I should have whacked the American and told him to go to hell right then. But I didn't. Even though my hand has whacked others, because that's sort of unavoidable when you run with boys, it didn't then. The American didn't leave me, either; he took me into his black BMW.

That was perhaps where fear took the driver's seat, with me jumping into the car for inexplicable reasons. *Weren't we enemies from the start?*

In this small, warm treatment room, another string of key episodes, landmarks in my story, begin popping.

MAYBE THE AMERICAN and I were both marked by our encounter a couple of hours before in the legendary discotheque in the heart of Denmark's second-largest city, blocks away from the place Dahlia now called home. Maybe that was why we found ourselves in the BMW, speeding to a hotel to spend the night.

This spectacularly sunny summer had been a terrific time to visit Dahlia. I was on break from university and had come to see her after a few days at home with my family. My three-day trip to visit her was a reunion for us, and, just hours earlier, we'd decided to go dancing at Downtown. That was where I'd seen him—the American. He had stood out in his chic preppy attire—white Polo shirt and shorts against olive skin—a contrast to the badly dressed male crowd that defied rain and wind at any given time on bicycles. They were clad for weather, not fashion. With his undulating, Elvis-black hair and blue-blue eyes, everything about him was styled and in place—crisp, like a glossy snapshot of an all-too-handsome man on a yacht in a Ralph Lauren ad in fashion magazines. I couldn't help but find my way to the bar next to him.

"Tequila," I demanded, and left ample tips. Why tequila, when Danes drink beer? That was a terrible choice; it removed all discernment. But it worked. I didn't know how to flirt, but I did know how to be cool now.

He turned to me. "You tip well. You can't be Danish?"

I downed the shot, swallowing my surprise. Despite the chic un-Danish look, it hadn't occurred to me that he might not be native until that moment. Discernment was gone even before we spoke. Rolling my tongue into the best Canadian twang I could muster, I said, "I'm Canadian. And Danish." Pause. "You want one?"

"Sure. I'm from New York."

His eyes shone bluer than Mother Karin's, and lots of sculpted bodybuilding muscles moved under the white, preppy cloth. A quiver, not unlike the one Rune's pecs brought on, had me as I quaffed another shot.

The American banged his empty glass on the bar. His lips enthralled me. Thin, as if shaped with gentle strokes by an elegant pencil, in the color of red currants. *If I were a painter,* I thought, *that's how I would portray an artist's vulnerability to his muse.*

"I hope you don't do drugs," I said. Drugs were a foreign land my curiosity never had begged to explore. In fact, I was a vehement believer that drug users were losers, and up to this point, I'd had no trouble steering clear of them. If they were in Frederikshavn, I didn't know them. At UFT, I'd declined the occasional joint offer because I was going places and drugs wouldn't take me there. Drugs were never on my mind—except they were here at the bar with the American from New York, a place of grit, gangs, and corruption. That's the news we received in Canada about the big city, the city of many shadows, which hadn't yet transformed into a clean Mecca for yuppies, power-shopping tourists, and trendsetters from around the world.

Yet it was a place that obviously rocked, because the American told me all about it. In the glittering discotheque, New York City turned into a play I longed to see because the Ralph Lauren model standing before me created a scene of its nightlife and jazz bills, Italian pizzerias that made you wet, a wild mix of people, and beautiful women who called it home, not to mention the money that ruled it. New York City was the greatest city in the world, hip like a David Mamet play.

But first, the man's dark hand moved to cover a dry cough. "No, I don't do drugs."

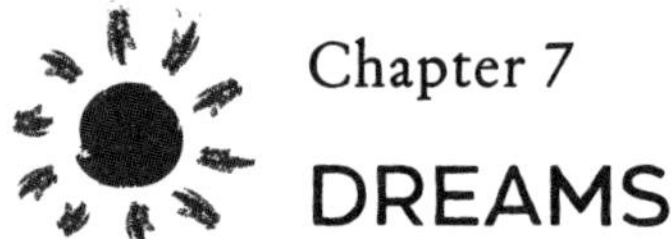

Chapter 7

DREAMS

Being a Dane studying at a North American university was outright unusual. I had to have rich parents who paid for it all, the American insisted. He was a trader with a seat on the Exchange, in Europe on business, and grabbing extra days to tour countries in a black BMW convertible. In social democratic Denmark, a BMW convertible bragged the status of a Learjet and was so exceptional he'd had to rent it in Hamburg, south of the border. That was nothing but impressive, and so was the Exchange, whatever that was, as well as his fluent French. He was almost a decade older than me and not tall, but he spoke about contemporary jazz like I would tell the stories I'd forged on my yellow typewriter.

Even in the haze that was setting in from more shots, the American drew me into his vortex. He was altogether different than the ruffled crowd of guys here and in Toronto, who always looked like they were coming or going to a soccer or hockey game. He was one big, enormous magnet, the size of the universe, and if I'd had the combined resistance of a heavenly and earthly army, he'd still have sucked me in, tequila or no tequila. I had no choice but to fall for him.

The flashback switches to the hotel where we stayed. It's mostly hidden in the haze. Only two backs turned against each other in a king-size bed stand out as contours from the night.

The following day, the American dropped me off at Dahlia's address. We exchanged nothing but a faint goodbye. Injuries and hangovers made us both reticent. He took off in the black convertible, going somewhere incredibly cool. The world wasn't a small place yet, and I never expected to see the preppy American again.

Fear could have stayed in the haze. I wouldn't be on this massage table with curled toes and anal pain had fate not intruded on free will.

The following day, Dahlia and I were at a local snack bar, filling our hunger, when the magnet as big as the universe showed up. He wore dark shades, a look to kill, and smiled at me. Before I knew it, I'd packed my bags and ended up in Copenhagen with him for three days during the best summer in Danish memory. It was as if the incident on the beach had never taken place—or perhaps the memory of it sought shelter in a hidden corner inside me. The will of fate was no match for my will, or maybe, just maybe, sometimes there is a blueprint, a fateful, grand blueprint for our lives, and no matter what we do, we cannot escape it. The American was in my blueprint.

The following days, we spent time in outdoor cafés, where the American read currency exchange rates in the *Wall Street Journal* and drank lots of cold Tuborg, carrying on about Pat Metheny, the jazz musician whose Missouri-Brazilian guitar sound had inspired him to set up his own music recording studio. We talked about politics, and my UFT political science studies and Magnum's dinner travel blogs turned useful in fast moments when my voice joined the conversation, and he almost paused. I became a traveler who had a new skyline in view, and parts of myself I didn't know about were kindled, as if libraries of books inside me had suddenly come alive. I was magnetized. He was ever so different. His coolness behind the dark sunglasses was big and wide. Cocky, Danes would say, because having the biggest and best of lives and flaunting it went against all rules for Danish modesty.

Cockiness was a social sin—and a challenge, something to flip the cover off. In swift moments, my gut spoke like other Danes; no move to Canada could eviscerate my roots. Why would someone so hip, rich, and from New York City be sitting with Nette from the north in a café in Copenhagen for three days? This didn't make sense. Yet I was having trouble hearing anything but the avalanche of information coming from the American, whose name turned out to be Calvin.

On the night before his return flight to New York, a chance showed up. Our hotel room was quiet. The American had been lying motionless on a still-made bed for hours, and that was just un-magnetic. Unexpectedly, in the unlit room with pulled curtains shutting out Nordic evening light, I heard my gut speak. *It* and *I* both wanted out. I needed light. I needed air. I needed to explore and breathe. The American wanted to do nothing but stare into space and wouldn't respond to the suggestions I made. This wasn't the cool New Yorker who'd lured me to Copenhagen.

I missed my chance. Calvin suddenly spoke. He told me he'd find a bridge and jump off.

I scooted to his side, not fully understanding the brevity of his words, but knowing I had to help him see nothing was ever so bad that it begged that end. Cockiness and dark shades came off as Calvin narrated what ailed him.

But before he did, he asked me to look for surveillance cameras in the room and to peek through the curtains and report if any cop cars were parked outside. They could be undercover ones, with cop looks, crew cuts, and roving eyes that knew your mind before you did, he said.

Wow! In the stuffy hotel room, a scene change took place, as if out of *Goodfellas*, and it drew me in. I was intrigued. I was curious. I was twenty-one. I was also disappointed, but that was neglectable. The cover was flipped off as Calvin told me there was no seat on the Exchange. He wasn't a trader but a bartender, though he did have a degree in economics and French and had attended Berklee College of Music, the place that bred successful jazz musicians. He was in Copenhagen to collect a debt and had been driving around Germany, France, and Switzerland, waiting for those who owed him big money to get it together.

Earlier that day, in the morning, when he'd gone to make a call at the green phone booth in the main square, his cousin, who owned the bar he worked at, had told him that Mitchie had gotten busted. Mitchie was the bouncer who'd procured coke to Calvin. If Mitchie had gotten busted, the cops must be onto him also, in Copenhagen and back in New York.

He'd also made a call from a different phone booth to his girlfriend. She was street smart, with balls like a man, and had taped cocaine bags between her long legs a few times when the sweat on his brow was giving him away at the airport check-in. Since she had taken on transporting the cargo more than once, she wouldn't squeal. She wouldn't risk her senior position in a big bank.

He wasn't repentant—how else, he demanded, could he have gotten all the techno instruments and recording gadgets he needed? His family was half Italian and half Irish, and though his dad used to have a decent job in the city, that wasn't enough to feed a brood of kids they never should have had. They were losers in a well-to-do suburb, their peers all filthy rich kids with Ivy League–educated parents who helped their sons get into college and real careers. He'd gotten nothing from his parents, so now he had to grab what others had been handed. But the customers weren't paying up this time, and he had no muscle with him to make them. He'd spent all his dough driving around Europe, and the cops would get him sooner or later. Who wanted to be handcuffed and gang-raped in a US penitentiary? Drug dealing was a federal offense and carried long sentences now. Prison hell was where he was headed. He was turning thirty, and his life was over, so he might as well make it quick and find a bridge.

Calvin was still wearing the white Polo shirt and shorts, but the clothes were now wrinkled, the look lost. All effervescence had left the man who'd appeared like a Ralph Lauren ad hours before. I was still crouched on the floor next to him, feeling his story and not myself. The cool Ralph Lauren man had to be revived. He had to be given a reason to see why his life was worth staying around for.

Fortunately, one of Magnum's powers, his skill of optimistic confidence that persuaded and infected its surroundings because it was so large it was impossible to dodge, was also mine.

With this skill, I started stroking Calvin's curls. Then I counted all the reasons why the law wasn't waiting and why federal penitentiary wasn't his fate. Why a one-man show wasn't important enough for a transatlantic undercover drug operation, with spying devices scattered around the capital, to be underway in the final week of the national vacation that shut down the whole country and that cops, too, observed.

As I soothed his beautiful, Elvis-black hair, he allowed that if he lay low for a while, perhaps things would settle. I heard him say I might be right. Copenhagen cops couldn't be bothered by a single maverick like him. His little brother had gotten busted for dealing in New Jersey a couple of years ago, but had gotten off on a technicality. Maybe there was a technicality he could claim, too.

Under my strokes, the wrinkled, white-dressed body uncurled and relaxed into the mattress. A while later, it rose from the bed and headed for the bathroom, grabbing a green bottle on the way.

I closed my eyes and smiled. Movement indicated the crisis had passed. My Magnum power had worked. Maybe we could head out soon, into the city I longed to get to know.

"You want one?" Calvin appeared in the bathroom's doorway with a pen stretched toward me.

"What for?" *Does he want me to take notes?* Yes! I yearned to bring this narrative alive on the keyboard that had replaced the typewriter months before. How did he know?

"You want some blow?" Calvin nodded toward the bathroom counter, which was visible behind the open door. "There's a line laid out for you." He moved the pen in my direction, and I noticed then that it wasn't a real pen. The moment stayed fixed in hotel space, as if a camera had zoomed in on the gutted, empty blue shell intended to be used to inhale the white powder. I declined but surrendered to accepting that Calvin did drugs. He both did and dealt drugs, in fact. But he made it seem like that was what winners did.

Seduction comes in many versions. Sometimes you can't blame anybody but yourself.

And maybe a pen.

While Calvin drank Tuborg and snorted into the night and the outside turned dark for a couple of hours, I came alive with the details he shared from his life in Boston in the 1980s, a time when party and coke were king. He'd checked out of Berklee after running into Sam, a tough, Nordic-handsome near giant with Finnish roots and a large personality nobody could outdo. He owned a gym and benched more than anyone else, steroids or no steroids. When he downed vodka, you couldn't tell. It might as well be water. He took a liking to Calvin because he scored lots of women in his part-time job as a shirtless bartender in a hot nightclub. In a swift sidewise motion, Calvin became co-owner of the gym and joint host and dealer of a lucrative business that turned the back room into a hot spot for parties. Their back room deals included trust fund crowds with monkeys on their back and rolls of bills to cover deliveries, local cops who liked clean blow, politicians, a couple of music pop stars, and known athletes who all liked a great party. According to Calvin, everybody was doing blow in the eighties, and there was no better place than their gym. No one wanted this party to end.

When the lines ran out, Calvin finally pulled me into his wrinkled white clothes. We hadn't touched since the spiky rush cut my back. Now we did. This time, Calvin stroked *my* hair.

"You are beautiful," he said, a grimace twitching his face.

Much later, I learned that's an inevitable shit-grimace. You stare, and you grimace; that's how coke works. But right then, Calvin called me "baby" and told me he'd always dreamt about someone like me. I was like a wild horse, he said. Must be the lanky, muscled legs that were anything but petite and maybe a glimpse into my heart, where horses roamed because their bodies moved like smooth-flowing ocean. I didn't need coke to feel high; Calvin was all the party I needed. Then he showed me other things I didn't know about.

For the next many hours, I learned about the lust that came with coke, and I learned some of what had turned Calvin into a sex expert. When we woke up, we called it love.

Calvin hurried packing because the plane was taking off. But he wanted more of me. Soon. He asked me to come to New York.

I agreed. How could I not?

BACK IN TORONTO IN a new year of studies, Calvin's face jumped out of the pages I tried to read. Weeks later, I found myself on the Upper East Side in a place called Cantina, a margarita before me on the bar, a huge TV screen with

American football playing behind me, and Calvin on a stool next to me. It was another scene, and it was called "doing the New York thing." I didn't know it, but in not too long, the TV show *Friends* would be happening just south of here in the West Village. For the first time, I tasted a margarita. Calvin lit a smoke. I felt the beat of the city in and around me, and cool was no longer just pretend.

I also felt engaged, a vibe of its own. Calvin still hadn't kissed me, not here or in the airport when he'd picked me up an hour earlier. But in the call that had me use up my student budget and book an air ticket to New York, he'd stunned me, and I suppose himself, with words that filled the landline between us: "I think I want to marry you."

His tone was void of cocksureness, and maybe that's why, after just three tries, I got that it wasn't a pickup line to a Danish girl going to a high-ranking Canadian university. Out of nowhere grew a desire that pushed everything aside and had me wanting to marry, too. Marry a cool New Yorker by the name of Calvin. This was an entirely different dream than that which had brought me to North America. I was young. I was foolish. I was following my blueprint.

That blueprint is energy set in motion when your first cry hits the air outside your mama's womb; it's handed to you by your soul as you enter Earth. It is a GPS for your life, your purpose, and your potential. By way of a subtle direction you don't know but do know, blueprints give us what we are meant to be. They do not have a rigid structure, but they do have flow and offer ample opportunity to make right or make wrong. Just like an architectural blueprint, the building you end up with depends on the builders who help bring the drawing to life. A bad plumber can play merry hell with your direction in the blueprint. Hooks in the wrong place can thwart its execution.

Away from Cantina and margaritas, back under Lynn's caress and Morfar's presence, I suddenly get how my blueprint has freedom all over it. I see blue lines defining the yearning that has motivated me since I was but a baby scooting down the stairs to free myself from a crib upstairs.

But on my way to freedom, I got lost in a blind spot called Calvin.

BACK IN THE THERAPY room, Lynn's voice snaps me back to real time.

"Take yourself off the hook, Nette. You were young, foolish, and you made mistakes. That's all right. You repair them and move on. It's just life. Don't make it more than that." She stops while the north pause happens.

Morfar knows I need more. "It's on them, *Nettepige*. It's on them to fix their soul-unhappiness. You can't ever fix your mother's, and you can't make up for it by fixing Calvin's."

Quietude is all there is while Morfar's words settle. I realize he knew much more than repairs and driving. Morfar knew presence; it was something he and Mormor brought when they saw, heard, and embraced their little granddaughter in ways only wide love and acceptance can do. It's a superpower, and it is also a strong blue line running through my childhood. Blueprints are nobody's responsibility but your own, and that is a tough thing to accept when you are very young, and someone is screaming, "I want to kill myself," and you don't know how to make it stop. But sooner or later, you have to realize that it's not your blue line but theirs. It's theirs to fix. Morfar knows so.

If only I'd had this direct line to him in the next recall at Cantina. But I didn't, and once more, I let another storyline seduce me.

"I'M GOING UP THERE. You wanna come?" Calvin's voice lured me.

"What's up there?" I forced a casual tone, hoping it wouldn't betray how little I knew.

"One Hundred and Sixty-Third Street." Calvin got up from the stool. "Spanish Harlem. Home of spics and motherfucking . . ." He mouthed the last word while looking around at the New Yorkers at tables behind us. They were lost in drinks and conversation. *Coke* was the unspoken word his lips shaped. I nodded in agreement and not a little delight. A coke purchase in Spanish Harlem, a short subway ride from the Upper East Side, was something tourists and regulars didn't get to experience.

"It's not the safest place in the world," Calvin warned me.

We were heading toward the subway stop with a direct line to the street where he had his Dominican guy. A chill December afternoon and yellow cabs in NYC traffic greeted us, and I shivered in the cape Mother Karin had designed for herself when she still was sewing in the basement and eighties fashion called for bright maroon. Months ago, I'd saved it from a dumpster bag. I liked its brightness.

"The place's loaded with cops," Calvin continued. "They look for people who stick out like sore thumbs, you know, like you. Try to blend in. You really should be wearing black."

Even though I knew I shouldn't, I giggled. I was heading into an area loaded with undercover cops as a blonde in bright has-been clothes that wouldn't ever make her anything but non-native and whose only possible errand in the Spanish part of town had to be buying drugs, which carried a prison sentence no matter your nationality and age. But Calvin had invited me into his story and being part of it created effervescence in my gut. *No* was never an option, for me or for Calvin. I wanted our tale to continue.

At Cantina, Calvin had told me he almost hadn't picked me up at the airport after seeing me waiting on a bench, looking unattractive and unfashionable. The crew cut I'd had to get after a recent faulty coloring job had caused a Ronald McDonald hair shade was growing out, leaving my hair at a length where it bobbed and bounced not like casual curls of the early nineties but like a dumpy mess that made me look like a Midwestern tourist.

"A sure barometer for anti-fashion looks," Calvin explained. Maybe it was the eighties clothes that I'd brought to New York in lieu of jeans, but he insisted they made me look chubby. "How are you going to get ahead if everyone looks thinner and hipper than you?" he demanded.

Black clothes were invented because they made people appear slimmer, so wearing an outfit shimmering with brightness from another era and plumping up my appearance was a huge turnoff.

Even so, he had come up to me on that bench, and we had left the airport in a shiny new Volvo. But I wasn't listening to the reel of details about the sleek black thing carrying us into Manhattan, to Cantina, because I was listening to my gut suddenly screaming, *No!*

This wasn't the reunion I'd had in mind for us. His girlfriend was supposed to be gone. Back in Copenhagen, Calvin had told me he was breaking up with her as soon as he returned to New York. But he hadn't. The car had been recently leased in her name, and she still lived across the street from his apartment building.

As I processed this news, Calvin turned on the radio, and the *No!* faded because Frankie Goes to Hollywood jumped into the seats with us. The naughty beat of "Relax" had Calvin doing drumbeats into the steering wheel while the melody of men, leather, chains, and controversy bounced off the Volvo's luxury seats. At that moment, Calvin's dream of becoming a recording pop star seemed as real as the bridge we crossed, and a zillion lights made the city look like a star, brightening the whole world. I forgot everything but the two of us together on a tryst in New York City.

SPANISH HARLEM WAS LIKE every scene in every movie about drugs and drug deals, but now I had my own recording of it. Our storyline continued on in Atlantic City, at the bottom of the New Jersey shore. After the coke pickup in Spanish Harlem, my fiancé wanted to get out of the city, away from cops. The blinking casino we entered near the boardwalk was a place of no joy, only tight faces, tense, wearied eyes, and cigarette smoke—billows and billows of smoke, as if all of China was on fire. Calvin wanted to do a round of blackjack and get free drinks before heading to a motel for the night. I stood by, watching, but couldn't stand the atmosphere.

A few drinks later, our date continued in an inexpensive motel room.

This time, I knew what Calvin was offering when he extended a pen case my way. I declined. Calvin grabbed a beer and took a seat in the room's only chair. I lay down on the bed and listened while he narrated the night away.

Daylight had arrived by the time Calvin moved to the bed. We pulled off our clothes, and he showed me once more the appetite that blow brought. Much later, before I closed my eyes to find sleep, a rare delight took hold of me. Calvin had, with his muscled arms wrapped around me, told me he loved me.

"I really, really love you," he'd whispered. His words were like a big, sweet cherry the size of Jupiter.

THE MOMENT I HAD foresworn happened when we woke up and Calvin decided to shower. A few lines were left on the bathroom counter.

"You want one?" He peered through the shower curtain. "Let's make it special for you. You do them all. You do the rest."

"All right," I replied. Calvin wanted to do something special for me. And he loved me. Discernment never got a chance; I accepted the pen case he handed me and bent to do the move I'd seen over and over by now.

As I moved to the bed, an acrid taste saturated my throat. I grimaced. But in seconds, a warmth penetrated my body and mind, like the best day of summer, where everything is possible, and life is a joyride you master. Except not even that did justice to the sensation overwhelming me on a bedspread in a cheap motel in Atlantic City while my fiancé showered off his own coke night. Every cell of my being felt the sensation of greatness—not a singular sensation of greatness but a greatness felt by several trillion parts of me.

Next, the lust arrived, a grand greatness all on its own. My mind and my body wanted to screw the whole world, and even that wouldn't ever satisfy the insatiable desire that had my crotch burn with a want so absolute that any cock and sex act I could imagine would be welcomed in those wrinkled motel sheets.

When the lust waned, I got up and did another line, and then another. I was beginning to like blow. And I was beginning to give myself away to something with no conscience, something with an infinite appetite for souls.

FAR AWAY, BACK IN the treatment room, I wish for a rewind button. I wish to freeze the motel moment and do a retake. Any retake, as long as it steers me clear of accepting the pen case and bending over to do a line that didn't stop there.

How many coke virgins did he have? How many of us were there? These are sudden, new thoughts that arise as I recall the start of our relationship.

"Your grandfather says to trust yourself. Trust your instincts. Don't blame yourself. That won't make a difference," Lynn carries on. "The powerless must take power from others. That's why you were broken in. Now, you have a chance to retrieve your power. Find your way back."

Who stole his *coke virginity?*

"The prison guard is sucking the life out of you. Your husband's taking all you've got. And he won't stop. Leave the prison, your grandfather insists."

It's as if Morfar is sending memory reminders to help me spot how I've built my own walls. I don't want to revisit any more of those pages I've razed from memory. I want to go back to feeling beige, to feeling nothing. The room's soft darkness holds me while I resist.

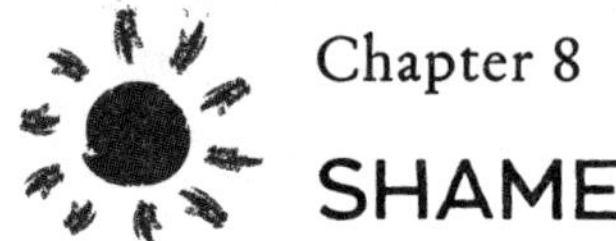

Chapter 8
SHAME

Break time is over. I can resist no more; I'm here to get unstuck.

The flashbacks continue.

THE FIRST DATE WITH my fiancé turned into countless more. I was in my junior year at UFT, and the Greyhound bus ride from Toronto took only ten hours, so I visited him every few weeks. My visits always followed the same mold: After the foil package was procured from 163rd Street, we found a bar with a good bathroom and hung out for drinks. The city was beating its beat: Skinny people in black with impressive CVs and lives stood next to us, also drinking and heading to the bathroom, and music and loud voices were participating, too. New York City was one big party, and I was in it.

Calvin lived in West New York, a handful of blocks in New Jersey that faced the skyline of Manhattan, and so almost in New York. Close enough to claim that he lived there, he explained. My fiancé was from the State of New Jersey, not New York—to many East Coasters, a contrast of kitsch vs. cool. And it turned out he *almost* had a dual BA in economics and French. He was just a few papers short of graduating. During my first visits, Calvin's impressive life modified, but how could I object? We were doing the New York thing.

On the sixteenth floor, in a large studio apartment with a white couch and a wall of synthesizers and recording instruments, the party continued. This party didn't differ much from the motel room in Atlantic City, except that Calvin used the kitchen counter to line up rows. He had a canister of empty pen cases; I was free to choose one. I did. Then I lay down on the futon in the corner while Calvin moved to the couch, each of us feeling the coke greatness in our own way. Calvin drank, and I didn't. Calvin narrated, and I listened.

While I was hosting several trillion parts of me feeling great and waiting for sex to happen, my fiancé's slow, frozen narration advanced down a road I was learning to dread. He started out bragging about the snowboarding trip he was planning to the Rocky Mountains, followed by the demo tape his sister, who worked at a major television network, was giving to some executive eager to hear his guitar tunes. Her husband was the VP of a big radio company, so Calvin had all the connections he needed to make it in the music industry. He had the talent, obviously. Everybody knew he was born with contemporary sounds in his bones, and it was just a matter of time before stardom was his.

With his inevitable fame established, the slow softness in Calvin's voice located a different pitch, the piercing kind that couldn't be ignored. The night shifted into his self-loathing overtaking the apartment, leaving me motionless on the futon.

Life sucked, Manhattanites and their fakeness sucked, people with Ivy League degrees sucked, Wall Street sucked, and his family sucked. They were greenhorns with no class who lived to survive and shop on Route 18, a place of inverted coolness. And he was nothing but a piece of shit who had no right to live. He was thirty-one years old, had no career, and was bottom-feed to the people who ruled the world's finances. Affirmative action had ruined his chances, and being a nobody sucked more than anything else. Why continue? The studio had a balcony, and sixteen stories was a good jump that would eviscerate the nobody in him. No one fucking cared. People cared only about themselves, and no one gave a shit about what happened to you.

Defying the brain freeze that bade me to remain on the futon, I got up to show Calvin some people did care and life could be different. He let me touch his hair, lightly. I stroked it until the pitch settled into something less dreadful and the balcony wasn't mentioned again. Sometimes, other things were mentioned—something involving an altar boy and a priest and, later, also a coach. And a red-eyed father who screamed and assaulted two young brothers in the downstairs bedroom that used to be a garage when he got home at 3:00 a.m. from work in the city and a few bars along the way. Nothing else needed to be mentioned because, between my hands, I felt the ache of a young boy who just wanted to play his guitar, for in his fingertips lay a universe of untold music he must bring to the strings like wind must blow and blackbirds must sing.

But the world had other intentions for him. Over and over, it proved so. When these things happened in the sixties, his mother couldn't make waves at church or at Catholic grammar school because she had five other kids to think of. She couldn't raise hell about the unmentionable things that everyone knew was going on. This story has been told a million times—and why the world doesn't change it, I don't know. Though I was still young and foolish, I did know a trauma was more than the nasty transgressions by a man-in-cloak or other adult. The deeper trauma was how your world responded—or didn't respond—to the misdeed.

A long arm on a couch behind you or card games after

dinner are measures against many things, and if given that, no one needs to find a way to dull the shame eating you up. When shame moved to own Calvin after Pa screamed, "You're a worthless piece of scum like all Irishmen and never should have been born," the presence of others would have connected him to the web of life where shamefulness can't grow roots. If shame is acknowledged—witnessed—it has no life. In the absence of presence, shame gets a free ride. This painful feeling of humiliation and inadequacy moves inside you, into the shadow place we all harbor, and becomes your new operating system. This invisible code breaks the connection to the other parts of you, and you feel and do things from a place of being a worthless piece of shit, someone who plunders to protect himself.

The sense of shame is god-awful, and you try to ignore the dishonor of what happened and of not being connected to your untold music—to who you truly are. But shame is a master, an emotion with no limits and no mercy. Day and night, shame owns you. You find ways to circumvent this operating system, even if only for short minutes on a couch with a line up your nose. You are simply seeking shame relief. Your appalled soul is screaming, *No!*—but you can't hear it because you are drowning in the misery that comes when you have lost touch with your destination in the blueprint. But all the while, that soul wants you to be happy and is working on getting you back on track, watching for a break when misery will become too much, and change will come along.

As I stroked Calvin's hair, I accepted the fact that the long lines on the kitchen counter were nothing but a phase for me. They weren't my destiny, even if they brought greatness to several trillion parts of me. Shame didn't own me as it owned my fiancé. I was still planning on becoming a journalist who wrote from foreign outposts to make a difference. Perhaps, if I stroked Calvin enough times and told him he wasn't a nobody but a somebody with potential and genius, with a signature sound and such a way with numbers that he could do dances around anyone at Lehman Brothers, I could uproot his shame. I could help upgrade the OS.

I was young and foolish and not following my blueprint's main line as I tried being a spot where Calvin could hook into the web of life.

DURING MY TRIPS TO New York from Toronto, where I was finishing up my undergraduate degree, a much-needed remodeling took place. Though we were kind of engaged, Calvin wouldn't have me meet anyone he knew until I shaped up. He claimed you couldn't live in New York without rocking a hip look. I could only agree—because who wanted to be a barometer for anti-fashion standing in a bar in the Village with her fiancé next to crowds of Manhattanites? New York City was going to be my home when I graduated the following year, so I'd better start becoming New York cool.

Calvin outlined how I ought to look on a napkin from Pink's, where he still bartended. The goal, according to him, was to be a ten-pound-underweight clothing size and possess a jeans ass that belonged in a Calvin Klein ad. He was the New York guru, and I was the tourist, so I declined everything but low-fat items and learned how to do squats at the gym—lots of them. My golden hair got lightened at the hairdresser's, because more was always better. My chest needed more curves, so Calvin introduced me to padded bras, a craze of the nineties.

My fiancé knew a thing or two about padding, I found out. His V-shaped bodybuilder physique had enhancements different from the steroids that had helped build it back in his Boston days. He wore insert soles and triple sets of socks and only sneakers for footwear. They allowed him to cram rolls of paper into the heel area, adding two inches of false height—a boost he needed, because the world favored tall people. This was also why he couldn't ever have a real career, for that required loafers, and hell would freeze over before he wore a pair. Only naturally tall people could do loafers.

The only time Calvin didn't wear paper rolls and sneakers was during sleep. Nobody knew about his false height. Below the Polo shirt, he also sported a padding trick taught by Sam: a triple layer of washed-out shirts cut off midriff to give the upper body an appearance of more width. Width was power in the bodybuilding world and beyond, and Calvin needed that power because the world was competitive and had no mercy for the weak.

As I remodeled myself to fit into Calvin's cover story, I learned how Calvin had stretched, shaped, and enhanced himself, physically and otherwise, to become the handsome Ralph Lauren American I'd met in Europe. But it didn't matter that the American from Downtown was altogether faux. He had me hooked, both with his story and his potential.

Somehow, I got the look right. My jeans ass turned CK ad-worthy, and on a dreary day in March, Calvin and I entered city hall in Manhattan to stand before a Black female judge and affirm a vow to each other.

Everything about this day was bleak. I wore black, and Calvin's mood was as dark as my dress when he told me on the subway back to the studio, where he had prepared a big pot of red pasta sauce and a foil package from up there for dessert, that he couldn't believe he'd done this. He couldn't believe he'd actually married me.

His hands cradled his face as he spoke. I couldn't laugh, nor could I cry. To be sitting in a NYC subway and be someone your husband regretted marrying minutes after the ceremony was a sorrow too enormous to be captured in the language of tears or laughter. I just sat there, staring into nothingness, while the train shot up Manhattan and Calvin rued his mistake that was me.

The truth was, Calvin wasn't the only one having qualms. I hadn't mentioned the planned wedding day to Halfdansvej. They didn't understand why I was moving to West New York after graduating when I had plans for a master's in Canada. They certainly wouldn't ever understand us doing blow because drug use fell into my family's category of worst possible delinquency. Mother Karin and Magnum wouldn't ever understand that I was doing drugs short term because that was the price of love. I was a mistake for Calvin to regret, yet I was no less sheepish about whom I'd married. With good reason, this day hadn't involved a white dress and tux, two golden bands, and a guest list. I had concealed the March event from just about everyone, even my best friend, Marianne. She'd been privy to every one of my crushes since seventh grade, but I'd kept her in the dark about this big day.

That night, Calvin turned to me in tears. He'd been deceiving me, he cried, and was going blind with something he needed to tell me about. I was at his side before the initial tear finished its trail down his cheek.

No, he hadn't cheated. It was much worse. When the blue contacts were removed, there was no hint of the handsome Ralph Lauren American; his kinship was more to a young Al Pacino—eyes like the darkest marbles against olive skin. I accepted this change. How could I not when he narrated how he hated his very brown eyes because they were a dime a dozen? If he weren't going blind from continually wearing his fake eyes, he'd never have told me. He'd rather go to hell than admit to the world he hadn't been born with blue eyes.

No one deserved such self-hatred, least of all because of an unwanted eye color. Turning secret-keeper of the ways in which Calvin covered up the true version of himself—the man who had stood in summer-warm water next to me howling,

"I am free"—came naturally to me. With unspeakable ease, I locked myself into my husband's prison of shame and turned away from truth.

LYNN'S SOFT VOICE reaches me. "It's okay. Let it go."

And I do. That part is easy in the warm treatment room because it's as if the outside no longer exists, and I am submerged in a dark space with a Rolodex of memories, each with a pertinent reason for begging my attention. I observe each memory, and then I release it.

In the next recall, the date picker shows November 1995.

WE WERE IN OUR new apartment in Minneapolis. I had run into enough Minnesotans wrapped in snowsuits and remarkable layers of hats, gloves, scarves, and boots to know Calvin was right about Midwesterners being anti-fashion barometers. Standing over a pot of store-bought tomato sauce heating on the stove, Calvin declared he was a shark among guppies and he friggin' loved this place.

"This place" was a red-brick apartment building a short walk from the University of Minnesota campus and home to graduate students, their partners, and other low-income people. Our new abode, a one-bedroom, had seen many winters and showed stains of wear you couldn't ever combat. Calvin was in graduate school, and I, two years after graduating from UFT, was working my first real job. My husband's eyes were brown now, and I was wearing my beloved colors once more. We were career-building, and New York cool was in the past.

While Calvin poured a heap of pasta onto a plate, I looked at the double-paned kitchen windows next to me. Ice filled the space between the panes. Outside, snow, ice, and frigid temperatures dominated the world at all times. I didn't care to listen to Calvin as he nattered on about the teaching assistantship he'd just finagled from Groe and how the finance professor was trusting him to code financial algorithms into an Excel program. The Minnesotan chill was one of a kind, the kind that I didn't easily make friends with. I had become quiet, very quiet, most of the time.

I stared at the checkbook on the table. It was also new. Neither Calvin nor I had ever possessed such an adult item before. Since we'd moved from New Jersey, it had been on me to ensure incoming and outgoing amounts were in balance. My job as technical assistant to a VP in a medical company had thus far supplied the incoming with enough to cover the outgoing transactions. I was making it work—and Calvin's new TA job would be an appreciated income boost. Minnesota was good to us, I told myself often. This city had welcomed us by accepting Calvin into a top-notch Master of Business Administration program with special focus on IT, bestowing on him a chance he hadn't stood in New York.

"You got something if you got a cutting-edge master's like this one," Calvin reminded me frequently. Once his music tape had been rejected, foretelling stardom wouldn't come from a demo tape handed to a radio network executive, he'd at last finished his undergrad degree. Now, we were here. Though I hated my job and believed I was made for much more than editing the spelling mistakes of a VP of Information Technology, living here was the cost of leaving that other life behind.

Calvin insisted that I enroll in IT classes because everyone was dropping mainframes and going computer and internet-crazy. And the *intranet*, had I heard of that? That was the new Klondike. I needed to do my part—get on this boat ride and make a lot more money—because the new technology was an opportunity second to none. There'd been no other fucking time in history like this; opportunities abounded, and we were in on it, Calvin told me.

I said nothing but tried to listen.

We were doing well in our new life. Yet I wanted to forget it all.

I GET IT, MORFAR. Oh, do I get it. I see the bricks building the prison walls and my hands on them. And if I don't, the next memory is a helpful reminder.

MONTHS LATER, WHEN THE evening programming classes my boss approved were completed, a familiar sound knocked me out of sleep. The spot next to me was empty. We had recently moved to a place in Uptown with a pool deck and an unobstructed view of the downtown skyline, subsidized by Calvin's new programming jobs.

"I can't do it. I can't cocksucking do it."

The shrill sound of despair made me sit up. Calvin's computer and desk, where he flushed out the magic of technology, were also in the bedroom, in the corner.

"They're expecting it tomorrow, and I can't fucking figure it out. It's a disaster. I'm gonna get fired. I'm gonna get found out. They're gonna know I'm a fucking fraud who lies about everything on his résumé."

Calvin dropped his face in his hands and rubbed and rubbed as if despair were a severe irritation on his skin. He had been banging on a computer in a bedroom for months, starting in New Jersey, where we'd gone to live with the Flannerys while Calvin attended the state university nearby to finish his undergraduate degree and I worked a temp office job. Night after night, he'd broken into one computer after another to learn its operating mechanisms. After we'd moved to the student apartment in Minneapolis, he'd continued staying up late into the night to figure out new software solutions for Professor Groe. These days, he no longer slept.

Calvin's brown eyes were red-rimmed by a different lure now: He had hooked his brain's unusual way with music and numbers to technology and found his stardom. Though it wasn't my dream, I was thrilled for my husband—thrilled he was finding success, thrilled because technology was like a shelter, a safe place, for him. And Calvin's connection to his brilliance was well timed, occurring during the boom of all booms, following Windows 95 and a "www." creation that unleashed a torrent of technology innovations that, with eyes of the future, could only be named revolutionary.

Calvin was right. Big, small, and transnational companies were releasing uncanny budget amounts to the promise technology offered, as if their survival depended on transforming the world into a place of user-driven screens with icons, pretty graphics, and software programs provisioning unknown needs. Enough was never enough, and that was why this was Calvin's time to strike gold, he reiterated. As such, he was giving it more than his best—still attending an accelerated MBA program, working two TA jobs for Groe, and, since the year had turned to 1996, also a full-time position at Sybase, a burgeoning tech giant. But Calvin's best wasn't always good enough. Several times a week, my sleep was cut short by wails in the bedroom. He needed someone to intervene.

"What's the matter?" I moved next to my husband and placed a hand in his mop of hair. He didn't shower much any longer. Baseball caps were a convenient invention for busy people like Calvin.

"I promised a prototype by tomorrow. Big-time Fortune 500 VPs will be present. They're expecting to see action, and I can't fucking get this useless code to work. I'm going to get fired. Gaston says the contract is in the bag if I show them the prototype. Do you think it's easy lying through your teeth about delivering something that hasn't been done before and then only having a few hours to figure it out, not knowing if it even can be done? I'm such a fucking loser. We're gonna lose everything if I don't get this bullshit to work. We should never have come to this godforsaken place."

Calvin buried his face in his hands. He had to get it to work, or he would collapse on the futon and not get up for days. Maybe never.

I knew he could do it. Because Calvin was brilliant. When it came to music, numbers, and now technology, he could do what others couldn't. I'd heard him play, and I'd watched him locate algorithms in the world around us, dark spots to others. So, in this moment, with all my honesty and heart, I told him how exceptional he was and how I knew if anyone could figure out a prototype in a just-released computer language in a few hours after days of no sleep, food, or showers, it was Calvin Flannery.

"You won't get fired," I added, still stroking his raven curls. "Come on, you're the best Sybase has. No one is doing what you're doing. You're way ahead of everyone with this coding. I know you can figure the rest out. You just need to calm down."

The Magnum power was still with me because Calvin sighed and returned to the screen. "Take a look." He pointed to the Java code that was supposed to marvel the executives into signing a million-dollar contract with the Minneapolis Sybase boss, Gaston. "I can't make it return a variable once a user has entered . . ."

I stood next to Calvin, watching unfamiliar cipher flicker across the screen. My own soul hated code; that was what the evening program had taught me, aside from giving me a certificate and enough insight to understand the gist of the coding principles Calvin was narrating.

A different yell soon erupted in the bedroom: "Yes, I goddamn got it. Look! I fucking bagged the elephant!"

Calvin did bag the elephant for Gaston, and the Sybase office grew, with Calvin and soon a whole team behind him. New contracts got signed, and Calvin had Gaston sign me on as well.

THE DATE TICKER TURNED to 1997, and I was making real money now, doing what I hated: working as a database administration consultant in a medical company. My soul refused stored procedures, the bread and butter of any decent DBA. Each day I entered the client site, I expected a hand to pull me into the Human Resources office—waving my résumé, asking how I came up with all these enhancements because I obviously didn't know a thing about databases.

"Lie, lie, lie . . ." I followed my husband's advice. There wasn't a day I didn't regret having ended up in my new job. But Calvin was probably right—everyone just wanted effing bodies, and there was no hand to ever worry about. In the Sybase training program I attended, there was a younger guy who'd bagged groceries the previous month and another guy who had a two-day tech certificate. The three of us were simply placeholders to fill into slots created by a tech craze gone amok. Gaston would hire monkeys for bodies if he could, my husband said, and the companies would accept them.

Loring was a café in an old industrial building opposite a city park a stone's throw away from our apartment, and with a style so completely its own, it felt like we were back in New York City. Loring had ice-cold beers, and every day after work Calvin recounted the latest from the office. Coding, the company, and software consulting were our new relentless reality, along with abundant disagreement. One cold beer for me and a few for Calvin, and it didn't matter that we were sitting next to filled bistro tables under glowing sunlight.

I might have been a lot younger than Calvin, and also in his vortex, but I had done a lot more than stroke his hair. I had been his sparring partner and given him a fight since the very first day we'd met by a bar. I had spoken my opinion, and I had not held back.

But that day, the fight within me died.

"I'm going to Toronto in two weeks," Calvin announced, grabbing the next beer the server brought by. He looked toward the greenery in the park. "A major Canadian client wants to implement an intranet. It's a great gig. It's the opportunity I've been waiting for."

"But . . . we are going to Italy that week," I protested.

"Come on," he said. "It's a once-in-a-lifetime opportunity. I can finally establish a name. The world's waiting for this intranet shit, and I'm in on it before anyone else. When will I fucking get another opportunity to make a real ordering intranet?"

As I tried processing all this, he slammed his beer on the table.

"Don't give me any friggin' grief. You're an ingrate who just married me to get a green card. And now you want to swoon over Italian men."

The big dream—becoming a journalist—was gone. Somewhere in the last couple of years, I'd given up on that. But our trip to Italy was my little dream, the dream that had kept me going evenings and weekends, trudging through books on computer architecture, code, and all the other terms that come with maintaining a high-paid consulting IT job when you can't even program a VCR.

For too long, there had been no time for anything but building a career I didn't want. But Italy . . . Italy had topped my bucket list ever since I'd read Luigi Barzini's *The Italians* at UFT, and I had been a little more alive knowing I was soon going to compare my own observations about the great people, the Italians, to Barzini's. Calvin wanted to go, too, to visit his roots in Sicily. We'd always agreed that traveling was sustenance—it was the morning coffee, the Barolo with dinner, the walk by the water. And now he didn't want to go.

"But we have tickets," I said weakly. "You said you would go for sure this time . . . you promised." But for once, I couldn't find opposition. There was nothing to defy. I knew Calvin. The gig had the final say. It was Toronto over Italy.

I got up from the bistro table and left before he saw the tears that came when the little dream that had held me together was snatched from me. I was going to live again, if only for a week, and now I was not. This was one sacrifice too many—one that changed everything.

The snatched little dream was also another missed opportunity.

MORFAR'S RIGHT. For a swift moment, before the next recall jumps in, I am back in the treatment room. *I really have to stop blaming myself.* For this and for folding my dreams into boxes shipped to a Copenhagen address, where they had no soil to become themselves.

The date picker rolls back to 1994.

MINNEAPOLIS WASN'T the first place we left New York for. After I graduated from UFT, Calvin insisted on making a clean start in my home country, where the government would subsidize his new life. We moved to Copenhagen, and after a few months on government assistance, Calvin persuaded a bank to lend us money to open a restaurant.

Quite like his parsimonious Italian grandma, who always knew where to find the cheapest plum tomatoes, Calvin's way with numbers and dishes cooked in mystery sauces didn't go unnoticed, and Danibank decided to bet on it. But even banks get fooled. A year later, the bet turned bad, and we were running through a rainy night to board flights to New Jersey, leaving unpaid rent, an empty restaurant, lines of creditors on our tail, and a mark of disgrace forever etched in my good name, even if our CPA advised us that this was just how business went. I had turned outlaw in my own home and had become "one of those people" whose name showed up on bad credit reports.

I hid in Minneapolis for a reason.

But I couldn't hide from shame; it was an amorphous being. I couldn't see it, couldn't feel it, couldn't hear it, but it stole from me. It stole any leftover yearning to pursue a dream that was just mine. The Canadian stories became a book from a life I didn't know, discarded in a drawer somewhere, just like the master's degree in journalism. Shame gobbled up dreams and didn't leave room for anything. Happy-go-lucky was no longer my nature, and I turned into someone who received career directions from her husband. I had no will not to.

Joining the dream of the man I'd married and struggling with stored procedures and Minnesotan chill was life at its easiest when you'd let yourself down as I had. I, too, lived with the worst feeling—that of soul screaming, *No!* That of being 100 percent off my GPS's course.

Is this where hate started?

I WALKED BACK TO our apartment from Loring, slogging across the pedestrian bridge with big cars racing below, hunched over as if hate was a collar of weightiness, worn but not felt. The little dream was all I had asked in return for shipping moving boxes to addresses where Calvin's dreams might thrive and staying there when they had flourished. This wasn't just another canceled trip. This was a betrayal. The kind from which you don't recover.

Months later, I packed another set of moving boxes, their labels affixed with a San Francisco address. We were going to live smack in Pacific Heights in an apartment with a years-long wait list because Cal had connections now. Young, urban IT professionals were already our friends. We were about to drop incredible layers of clothing and turn West Coast hip. Cal had been headhunted by the Cisco Sybase office for his web development experience, at that time akin to being, if not Columbus himself, at least an officer on the *Santa Maria*. Cal wasn't just exploring; he was helping to define this new world, in that the Toronto gig had led to him creating the first-ever intranet ordering system: Log on, select your purchase, pay, and get delivery. Four given steps today. But in 1997, Cal made history by providing a local sales force the ability to select and order their new vehicle on something called an intranet. With that, a universe of opportunities had arrived, and the West Coast wanted him. A reassignment for Cal's wife was part of the transfer package. We'd been out there a few times by now, and San Fran felt like home.

Cal stormed into the apartment one afternoon, interrupting the packing and our new life.

His brown eyes lined in red, he stammered out his new score. "I think . . . I think I just hit the jackpot."

I let the roll of tape finish its job along the top of another cardboard box and tried to recall whether there was enough tomato sauce left in the fridge for two.

"Which one?" I asked. "Powerball?"

"It's goddamn better than that. Paulie Pakalski thinks I'm God. He just moved to an IT director position at an even bigger Fortune 500 company. He's made me an incredible offer. I just had cocktails with him in Eden Prairie."

While I stacked the ready-to-move box, Cal's voice recovered its natural force.

" . . . independent contractor, and I can set my own hourly rate. Sybase pay is small nuts compared to this. We're gonna be rich! This is a fucking jackpot, I'm telling you. I've got Paulie wrapped around my finger, and there are more web projects than cocksucking sinners in church in the pipeline at this top 500 company. Nobody has done what I've done, though it's just a matter of time before every nasty Indian with a PC copycats me. We got to jump on this. Figure sixty hours a week times—"

"What about San Francisco?" I asked.

"We can't move now." Cal looked at me, not his laptop or phone. "I mean, don't you think I should take this opportunity? It can't go wrong, it just can't. It's now or never, while I still got game. Before cocksuckers like Harvard MBA types in the big consulting firms who don't add up to dogshit move in on this. This client is a behemoth, but once I get my foot in the door, these pussy Midwestern executives won't know what hit them. It's a jackpot, and I can't say no!"

That was how an "almost your dream" crashed. The annual pay figure Cal guesstimated bedimmed everything a West Coast yuppie life would offer us. On this sad day, Cal hit the jackpot, and shortly after, we moved boxes upstairs into a two-bedroom apartment with a terrace, rather than starting a new life in the Golden City.

Overnight, Cal changed from being a student programmer burning midnight oil to an independent project manager responsible for a million-dollar project. That's perhaps peanuts today, but it was big bucks in the late nineties. Coding was now left to the consultants, whom Cal contracted to fulfill the project deadline he had signed on for with his new client—then the world's largest company. As CEO of IService, he did what the big consulting firms wouldn't do: sign a fixed bid, which meant the project had to be delivered on time, or Cal would pay for extensions. Such a contract was a bit like an Atlantic City casino trip to tempt fate and fortune, except for Cal, it wasn't. Camels would fly, and oceans would bleed dry before he'd have missed the deadline. His grandma had owned a vegetable shop and survived the Great Depression with a surplus, and she'd taught him never to lose a penny doing business. There was only one option: making a million.

IService became the only company in the Twin Cities that delivered an IT project on time during the mad tech revolution. Our new investment account at Wells Fargo grew rapidly.

During daylight hours, Cal worked at client sites; this was followed by long hours in establishments in Eden Prairie, where he and Pakalski talked shop over cocktails. A lanky man with speech faster than Cal's, Paulie was a weak link at the top 500 company, my husband told me. Paulie had no tech experience. That was immaterial in the corporate world because he'd been hired to manage resources—people, computers, projects, same thing—but it's possible he was feeling as I still did about stored procedures: *What in the hell did I get myself into?*

Cal became his go-to guy, the person who told him all he needed to know to manage stuff he couldn't have pronounced the name of the day prior. The track of expenditure led to Paulie's desk, and Cal knew a trick or two from his dealer days in Boston—"Give them a freebie, and they'll come back for more." That approach worked; Paulie converted Cal's pitches into projects so immediately that they poured in too fast to count and fathom.

Aside from tracking project timelines, Cal's foremost task in life was making his customer happy so he never would look elsewhere. That was a sizable task, because Paulie had many whims. If Paulie wanted to take up shooting, he and Cal bought guns at Dick's and found a shooting range. If Paulie needed a new vehicle, they visited Suburban dealerships. If Paulie became a sushi aficionado, they frequented the best sushi bars in the Twin City area. And if Paulie wanted to go sousing—which he did most days—they went sousing. Thank heavens Paulie was a decent guy who only asked for a luxury car, not a blow job or something more wicked.

ANOTHER MEMORY SOUVENIR, dated 1998, shows Magnum making regular Sunday calls from the Peachtree apartment in Atlanta, where he now resided 180 days a year in his new position as US manager for the Danish concrete pipe machinery company.

I didn't tell him the toll building an IT empire was taking on me and his son-in-law; I only told him about the next project lined up, the figures in our bank account, and how I still struggled with stored procedures and the lurking threat of an HR hand on my shoulder.

Magnum let me know he was proud that I'd found my niche in Minneapolis. Once or twice, he admonished that Calvin could make time for a little fun for us. If you asked him, good times, not money, made the world go around.

Magnum was the only friend I had in America, and I didn't want to upset my confidant. I couldn't tell him how I cringed each evening when the sound of a laptop bag hitting the floor announced Cal's return from a long day of juggling projects, people, and deadlines, followed by sousing with Paulie. The name-calling started in the hallway before the apartment door was even thrust open, and I knew Magnum would have no tolerance for his daughter being called a slut, an opportunist looking for a permanent green card, and all the other things my husband shouted. Cal filled the kitchen with accusations because I was one of them now, the CIA who had stepped up their game in light of the development work he was forging. Now, it seemed, they were testing out poisons on spectacular brainchildren like him, and I was a part of it. It was my fault he was going to lose his hair to a contagion intended to defile and infect great people like Calvin Flannery.

I sighed and waited for it to pass, but I was always pulled into the vortex thrashing through our home. When Calvin began rubbing his face—vigorously, as if the CIA poison were searing his skin—no longer did I stroke the black gold. Instead, I stayed on a kitchen chair, frozen, as he ranted that he'd gamble the entire Wells Fargo portfolio on a bet sure to fail because I deserved nothing, I was a Scandinavian whore, and he should have listened to his mother and stuck to his own kind.

I wish you had.

Words have power, Magnum always said. Words are beings that don't leave but must settle somewhere. I didn't know where they went as I remained stuck to a chair, accompanied by the dread of spending yet another evening with my husband.

THE NEXT MISSED opportunity, I could *never* regret. From the treatment room or any other spot in the solar system, I could never regret that instead of leaving Cal, I asked for a baby.

The words struck like an unforeseen thunderclap when, rather unusually, we were together on the futon one wintry February evening.

"I think I want to have a baby." I was twenty-nine years old, the year had just turned 1999, and perhaps I knew I was unhappier than ever and needed a reason to go on. Perhaps there was a little soul waiting to live out her own blueprint.

My words spoke of a desire for change, and change came along.

Cal, due to an inexplicable universal law, answered that we *could* have a baby *if* I turned housewife. Any child of his would have to have the best. That meant having a parent at home, and he obviously wasn't going to do that job. Then he gave way to the staccato laugh that made me cringe.

Being a homemaker was the destiny of those *Frederikshavner* girls from my grade who had little aspiration or vision. Whose annual income I had beaten several times over now being that I, too, had turned independent IT consultant. Yet I agreed; no second thought needed.

It took me only two weeks to recognize the presence of life inside. My pregnancy was a slam dunk.

We were both elated. Truly.

In the final months of an entire century, November 1 arrived. Of course, the little soul couldn't have chosen any other day to descend. In the Lutheran tradition, November 1 is just another day. But for centuries before the Roman Catholic Church ripped this day off its pagan rivals and called it All Saints Day to honor all holy people in heaven, the day was long celebrated as the Feast of Samhain or All Hallows Day in pagan societies. It marked the beginning of another dark-light cycle, a new season of darkness that would continue until the light of summer arrived. Pagans understood that darkness inevitably carries the light, that darkness and light unite and dance in perfection, and that dark silence conceals whispers of light beginnings. This was a great moment to celebrate, and also a perfect day to be born when you're a little soul destined for the marital chill of two warring, wounded parents.

Change had come. Swiftly, like everything in the final years of the century, I was a mother. On my chest lay the most beautiful little thing, already suckling, her long, finely curved lashes something I'd known before. Calling it love was much too trivial; I was her mother, and for her, I would do what I wouldn't do for myself or any other person. For this little, precious being, I wouldn't merely move a mountain—if I had to, I would move a world.

Then and now, alongside Lynn and Morfar, my little girl is something that brings incandescence, making darkness retreat whenever she comes to heart and mind. This sensation has one name only: grace.

But Grace wasn't to be her name; it would be something even better. I'd never truly recovered from the letdown when Mother Karin didn't permit me to keep a lion in the bike shed on Friggsvej, and I wanted to name my baby Dandelion.

If you'd ever rolled down Kirseholt's meadows, sparkling with thousands of yellow flowers that purify the air, and you'd collected and twisted those flowers into little posies while feeling their sticky juice staining your fingers and smelling of Earth herself, you'd know each is a miniature sun whose nature is to bring radiance so soul-happy may thrive.

Cal vetoed the name. With a cackle. But he did agree to another name, an uncommon flower name closely resembling Dandelion. Although we settled on this other fine name, my baby will forever be Dandelion, the girl who changed the dark-light cycle in me.

The dark cycle hadn't yet retreated when the cell phone rang in the hospital room where mother and her newborn velvet bundle lay in fresh, white linens and bliss of new life. Cal stood by the bedside, inspecting Dandelion's nose for a bad bump he thought he saw, his finger sliding down the little bridge for confirmation.

"Come on, give it up. Why would she have a bump? And who cares about—"

My objection was cut short as Cal stepped to the corner to answer his phone. Why he answered, I don't know. He was getting sloppy.

"Where are you?" an agitated voice demanded. A female voice. And not his ma or sisters. "Why haven't you answered!" Its sound summoned up crazy-looking Glenn Close in *Fatal Attraction.*

My husband cleared his throat and responded with careful diction, "It's been a long delivery. I am with my *wife* and *newborn*—"

"I don't like it when I can't get hold of you," the voice screeched. "I have been calling and calling. I want to know . . ."

She had to be stupid, or perhaps she hadn't yet learned that a sure way to set off Calvin Flannery was by making him feel put-upon. That kind of behavior was guaranteed to make him start shouting, just like he did that morning in the hospital room with his newborn swaddled in his wife's embrace.

"What kind of person doesn't congratulate you on your newborn?" I asked when the shouts ended. I already knew the answer, because she was clearly one of the reasons for the chill that had lain between us in the past many weeks. I realized now he hadn't kept his promise. She was still working for him, and he was still bonking her.

She could have him.

Cheating was one principle to which I would not surrender, and Cal knew it.

"I promise," he said. "I will fire her. I will."

We checked out of Fairview Hospital and went home to the apartment overlooking the Sculpture Garden. Then, three months later, the scheduled move to the mansion on Long Island happened, and I started living with our baby in a geographical location I knew as well as I know streets on Mars. I was alone—no family, no friends, no husband—but even so, this new life beat growing roots in the state that had never grown on me. No child of mine was going to grow up in a state with no ocean.

Project timelines and Paulie kept Cal in Minneapolis except for occasional weekend visits to Long Island. Learning how to care for a baby's needs in a foreign place on my own took all I had.

THE RIGHT TIME, the time to truly ask for change, arrived five months before this very May day in Lynn's office, on our first Christmas in New York, the year showing 2000.

Dandelion was now a soft thing on wobbly legs, and I couldn't bear to think of her growing up with more holidays like this. I'd promised my daughter so much more than a dad doing coke in the basement of her grandparents' home Christmas Eve with two of his siblings while the rest of us sat upstairs next to a fake tree and no other Christmas spirit. Cal was in touch with the white powder again. A line up his nose superseded being a good parent any time of the day.

Never again, Dandelion. No more Coke Christmases. What I accepted for myself, I would not accept for my daughter.

A few months later, I found myself in Lynn's office.

LYNN'S SOFT VOICE reaches me through the warm darkness. "Your grandfather is supporting you through this, and you will be all right. I see him laughing again, because he loves you so very much and because he knows you can do this—leave the prison, get a divorce."

After a pause, her hand lightly touches my shoulder, and I know the reading is over. I'm back in real time.

Minutes later, I am on a sun-swept sidewalk, looking to the sky and thanking everything above and below me. The only person who could get through to me, who sees past the shiny cover of a story and won't ignore that I am not doing fine and don't know how to change it, Lynn Leclere brought into my presence. Morfar has opened my eyes to the pages of a life I've been covering. He has made me see why I am stuck in a story I never intended. Life is suddenly full of opportunity.

Either force, gratitude, or joy has me dancing on the sidewalk while Long Islanders zoom by. My shadow is cast on the sidewalk. I am getting unstuck. I am turning myself free. I am filing for a divorce.

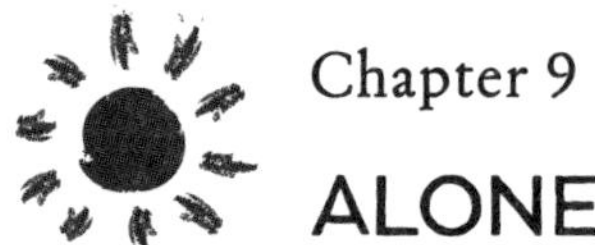

Chapter 9
ALONE

The pillow is lime green, the color of my newfound freedom. My face is buried in it while tears soak the lovely hue I chose as soon as I moved into the new home up the Boulevard from the mansion. The summer of 2002 has been awful, and not at all the way life was supposed to be. Two years after I, sitting on a yacht surrounded by exuberant July Fourth millennial celebrations, woke up to being stuck in a story and marriage that never was my dream, I am not the least bit happy or content.

Mere weeks after my session with Lynn last May, I filed for a divorce. Though the notion of amicably divorcing Cal was the equivalent of asking for a cordial war in the Holy Land, the divorce almost became a simple matter. In very fast motion, I got out, and I got Dandelion because Cal got to write the divorce agreement. One town over and yet a world apart from the town of mansions where I never met a single resident, I found a regular house filled with windows and light and a backyard with a swing set and neighbors that, no kidding, bring over apple pie and shovel your sidewalk. A new chapter started in this sanctuary.

The anal pain and other woes that brought me to see Lynn Leclere a year ago scrammed as soon as Dandelion and I moved into our home in Seaside, and the dominant color in every room became lime green because Cal had always vetoed this color. I started making friends, and I started pursuing a pragmatic dream to become a high school teacher to support my toddler and myself. Around this time, Sister Sallie, who at the time was working in a kindergarten and lived in an apartment in Frederikshavn with her two sons and, most of the time, her boyfriend, Leif, asked me to return to Denmark. Never for a second did I entertain this request, even though Cal didn't mind our daughter leaving for a different continent.

Little Penis's reaction to the divorce news was neutral. Mother Karin's response was not.

"Why are you doing this? Now I got two divorced daughters!" she yelled. Then she issued a counsel to stay with Calvin and just avoid having sex. She took to her son-in-law once he started bringing in a noteworthy paycheck in Minneapolis, and she also admired how he learned Danish in less than three months and code overnight.

Magnum, on the other hand, understood my desire to leave Cal but remain in the US. Somehow, this great country has turned home for him and for me.

At first the good days were many, because a new sanctuary with walls and cabinets to fill, a neighborhood to fall in with, and hope and possibilities to uncover had me jumping out of bed each morning, longing for the day to start. The kitchen with the wooden floors, framed by windows and a backyard terrace, got to witness Dandelion and me trying out dance moves with Sade's soulful tunes turned up loud. I even went out with some men at first—but I dumped dating in no time, because I didn't need anyone interfering in my new chapter, least of all someone who carried ex-husband traits.

And yet bad days also dropped by. Breaking up even an awful marriage begets grief. Giving up on a life after finding yourself unable to make it work and leaving a story gone off isn't always as easy as it sounds. But that's not why I am soaking my lime-green companion just now.

Why didn't I just let Cal be in his new life? Why have I let myself get collared into his world again, a place that includes a Chelsea rooftop apartment and a bigger Sea Ray? Why do I answer when he calls? Why do I shoot into the city with Dandelion in the back seat when he hasn't slept for days to help him calm down and fall asleep? Why in heaven's name did I ever agree to a Thai meal on the most scorching day of summer, when even a fool knows that's a day ripe for food poisoning?

After that meal with her dad in a nearby restaurant, both Dandelion and I woke up late at night. She vomited, and I sprinted for the loo. The next morning, her chubby body scooted off to find new games in her bedroom next door, but cramps made me curl up and general awfulness had me stay in bed. Not just for a day or two, but an entire summer.

Now, though fall nears, my body is still writhing from a cramp that starts in the gut and spreads to the rest of the body in an attempt to cleanse itself of something that needs to come out but won't. The anus woes are back, along with reoccurring loo calls and nits in the stool that the gastro doc dismisses but gives me Vicodin to help me unmind. Mask the pain, ignore the root cause—that's the prescription. But I cannot, because my life is ruled by the exhaustion and apprehension that follows a summer in bed and an intestinal bug that just doesn't want to pass. And Dandelion, my sweet velvet thing who hugs at all hours and has me read her stacks of books aloud and do silly games with her on the floor, is on my mind all the time.

These days, Kathleen, the babysitter I hired when living at the mansion, is doing fun things with my baby girl. My legal status has changed, but I am still stuck. *Because who will look after Dandelion if I am consigned to a hospital bed?* No one. And that's an overwhelming thought, a monster apprehension, that has me burying my face into the comfy lime-green ally and crying out a mother's nightmare: her child abandoned.

Unless you've been a single parent and only child living together—just us, always together, aside from a few hours a week while she attends pre-K—you can't imagine the bond that exists between us. We share time, space, love, games, and bed all the time. When I breathe, Dandelion feels it; when Dandelion laughs, her giggles are mine, too. She is dew, and I am morning; I am mist, and she is daybreak. *Wonderful* is a meager word to label our closeness. We are a unit, a mother-daughter corps that thrives together and in balance. And I am so sorry for what I've just done to her in the kitchen downstairs. So sorry, because it's been this way for a while now.

Dandelion appeared minutes ago in the bedroom, stretching her arms toward me and asking for a hug. She's a tall toddler, going on three, with light, bouncy hair and Sicilian brown eyes that miss nothing. Not tears on lime green, certainly.

"Mama," her voice rang like silver bells. "What this?" In her hand lay some object.

Even with my back turned, I sensed her eyes fixed on the damp pillow. But I didn't move my head to look. I am no longer the mother who promised to move a world for my baby daughter. I've become someone else, someone who can barely move her own body and is struggling with the demands of motherhood. "Can't you just shut up?" I sobbed. "Not now."

The exhaustion has turned me into someone who acts nothing like the mother Dandelion and I both knew. And no tears or promises to have a picnic in bed can rid me of the regret I feel for having spoken to her that way.

After a few seconds, I pulled myself up and moved downstairs to help my little girl find a bowl of cereal or something that could become a picnic and cover some of the hurt from a mother gone off. But my attempt didn't remove the new shade in the big brown eyes of my daughter.

Maybe I am also crying because, in these past months of change, I've avoided war with Cal but not with Sister Sallie. We are not speaking, and I remain furious at her after a bad day following the divorce.

Several months ago, when Dandelion was coming home from her first overnight visit with her dad in his penthouse apartment, the day turned really crummy the moment Sister Sallie took my call.

I had just picked Dandelion up at the train station in town. Letting my girl spend the night in the city made me anxious, since she wasn't yet old enough to cross the street by herself or change her own diaper. But a girl needs a dad, I know so, and so when Cal found a vacancy in his schedule, I let Dandelion go. Of course, he'd arranged for backup—I ought to have known. Sitting in my black Jeep Cherokee, facing the station platform where LIRR trains transport hundreds of family men clad in Wall Street attire back and forth to the city each day, I quickly noted a fair-haired little girl wearing pastel pinks and yellows and holding the hand of a young woman with admirable hair way down her back, a skirt so short she needn't bother, and lanky legs.

Why did he have to involve a girlfriend already?

The leggy woman suddenly stopped dead and unclasped her hand from the little one. The little girl swung around. I felt her puzzlement; she wanted to know why her new friend wasn't coming along. But her dad yanked her forward—abandoning the backup and any possibility of goodbyes and teaching my daughter it's all right to turn your back on people you play and sleep with. Teaching her to pretend not to know a person lingering behind, though she has fed and changed you. A simple goodbye would have cut it. But that was too much to ask of Cal.

Near combustion had me call my sister as soon as I flung the front door open. I spewed into the receiver, trusting the familial voice to support that Cal shouldn't have yanked our daughter away from the backup, let alone brought her into Dandelion's first night with him at his new address.

"It's not your business what Calvin does," Sister Sallie asserted. "He's Dandelion's father, and he's responsible for her."

That was her answer, an ocean apart from a response I trusted, and this added to the combustibility that had tailed me from the train station. I was expecting Sister Sallie to hold space for what I was feeling, because I was having divorce pangs, and she ought to remember those. During her own divorce, her son was snatched from her, and a court case required the unloading of a parental pension coffer to enable Magnum and a Danish lawyer to fly to Michigan to entangle toddler Cody from the illegal seizure by his dad. And when my former brother-in-law attempted to trick me into bashing my sister's parenting skills, intending to record it for evidence in court, I made sure he failed. Sister Sallie ought to remember something like near combustion surfacing from an unknown body well, settling just below the skin's surface from where this being sprang forth at the merest hint of more injustice. But she didn't.

"Exactly, he's responsible for Dandelion—but show me a person more irresponsible," I erupted.

"You want to control him. Let them explore their relationship. You're letting your anger get in the way. It's not conducive." Sister Sallie's recent social worker degree and textbook theories lent an unusual surety to her attitude. I didn't know where my sister had gone. And I didn't know why she wouldn't have my back. I'd had hers.

"You're saying I should let him expose Dandelion to a parade of girlfriends, taking turns kissing her goodnight? And let Cal teach her it's fine to dismiss them?"

"She needs to learn who her father is, not who you want him to be," she insisted.

"But . . . but she's two!" I protested. "It's my job to protect her. I'm her mother!"

"That's a construct. And you're always butting in where you shouldn't. Try something else for a change."

Sister Sallie had never gotten into a word battle with me before. That was altogether new. I couldn't hold back any longer. I behaved as if my emotional cruise control had moved from chill to explosive.

"Damn you! You're a turncoat, always first in line for everything, even disloyalty!" I retorted. "Why am I always the bitch with you guys? Why! *Why!?*"

I couldn't stop, so I did something we don't do in my family: I hung up on her. And that's how our cold war started.

Why couldn't Sister Sallie acknowledge my right to anger, even if she believed I was breaking all textbook theories? Why couldn't she give me a moment's liberty to express the accumulation of feelings behind the story that was Cal and me?

I feel so alone. So alone with the divorce pangs and raising Dandelion.

My new life wasn't supposed to be this way, and yet it is. The divorce has not healed anything. Being let out of prison has changed nothing. I am still ill. I am still soul-unhappy, and this life is simply a new version of something old.

And that's the real reason I am crying on the lime-green pillow.

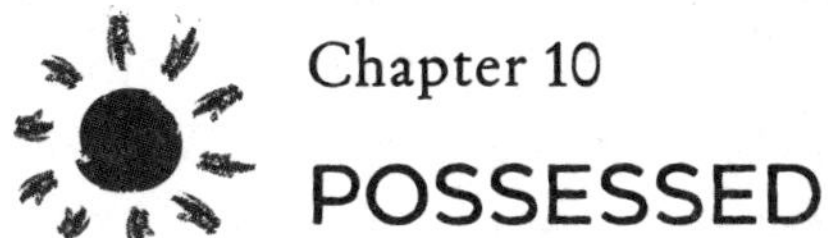

Chapter 10

POSSESSED

I am standing in the light-filled kitchen—knuckles clenched, possessed. The wrath within me wants out. I have turned into a stark, mad mother who screams, "Why are you bothering me? You don't need a Clifford Band-Aid! Grow up! Why do I fucking have to do *everything!*"

Next, I pummel my hands into the wall with the might of Stonemason Lars, until a lucid thought warns me a broken hand won't make life any easier. I stop, and my wrath is assuaged for a while. Then I look down at my almost four-year-old girl. Her currant-red mouth is quivering, and although tears cover the fine sheen of her eyes, she can't yet cry. The thrashing female in the kitchen might lash out some more, and her body is stiff with fear.

I recognize the stiffness that wraps itself around Dandelion's heart in this moment. It's an instinctual stiffness born when the person who is supposed to protect you is the person hurting you. The little kitchen upstairs at Friggsvej witnessed screaming moments when big drops of milk spilled onto the carpet or when Sister Sallie didn't get that if you have five apples and eat two, three are left (she was as bad at math as Mother Karin was at teaching it). I know what vitriol hurled at you by a mother's killing voice feels like in your body. It freezes your heart and then your gut. If you're Sister Sallie, you sit tight and wait for the screaming to pass. But if you're Nette, your legs carry you out the door and downstairs.

Dandelion doesn't run. She has nowhere to go. No amount of forgiveness can ever make right what I am doing to my little child. But I try. Unlike Mother Karin, I fall down next to my girl, wrap her into me, and I tell her how sorry I am. And then she cries. She cries into me while I whisper into her, "It's not your fault, *skattepige*. It's all my fault. You don't deserve any of this, and I am awfully sorry I yelled at you again." Then I squeeze her tight until we go find the Clifford Band-Aid that set the madness off.

But before we do, I open the cabinet above the stove, reach into it, and grab a plastic bottle. With the brown pharmacy bottle in my hand, I look at its small print, and I say, "*Fuck medicine*."

And fuck the doctors who won't listen to me. I've been hospitalized twice. The war with Sallie was settled when our parents arranged for her to come stay with Dandelion during the first hospitalization; a patchwork of babysitters covered the other stay. Both times, doctors filled me with cocktails of drugs to deaden the irascible way my gut was acting.

Now I am saying, *No!* to 80 milligrams of prednisone a day. The high steroid dose the docs are filling me with is way too much for my system. The roids have turned me into Mother Karin, and this must stop. I have become my own worst nightmare, duplicating the ordeal I was going to eclipse. Ancestral pain is carried over and lives within us descendants, and is ours to endure until someone is brave enough to face it.

That time is now. This has to stop.

A tear-streaked Dandelion holding my hand, a too-forgiving little girl, is my reason.

MDs are simply following protocol and a one-size-fits-all standard. Yet none of them are improving my symptoms.

They're as bad as ever. At night, I sprint up and down the stairs, looking for things to iron, and an overpowering quiver rises inside me, making me pound my feet into the hard floor of the kitchen as I move through the house. I either pound or I burst. And I rage. I rage like a lunatic Mother Karin tearing into walls in an apartment in Canada.

Many months have passed since I decided to trust doctors and accept their drugs, their solution to the medical diagnosis that Sister Sallie, too, received just before she ran off to sunny California. Drugs have worked for her, and the bad parts in her gut were surgically removed years ago. In me, however, drugs are not fixing anything; rather, they are nourishing the wrath, making it hurl even harder to get out. It's stronger and bigger than ever now, thanks to the trust I've put in medicine.

And I know better. More than two years ago, amid the divorce proceedings, a secretary called to relay the Crohn's diagnosis from the gastro MD I'd been to see. I needed to take a medication daily—forever, in fact, she added. I went to the pharmacy and took one look at the Rx insert. It was an easy choice then. I rejected Asacol and the long list of serious side effects. I said, *No!* to drugs, finally. A cover is but a cover, a fine veil on something ill or gone off below but never a healer.

Besides, prescription medicine is not how nature heals—and I am a miniature Earth, a microcosm of the macrocosm. Like the big being we call home, give me the right tools, give me time, and I will right myself. Because balance is what you, me, and Earth herself seek, and it is a natural law for all beings to seek the health of equilibrium. Nature doesn't break her own laws. Yet for some unfathomable reason, I have ignored what all of me knows and for the last few months have been trusting medicine to fix me and my gut.

Now, standing with a bottle of prednisone in one hand and a fair-haired little girl in the other, I suddenly know with all the might of my forefather, Stonemason Lars, that there is a better way to heal my inflamed bowels and their companion woes than what a flawed rule of medicine dictates. And I am going to find it. I am seeking balance, and that means I am seeking truth. I am seeking to let go of the untruthfulness I've navigated by. The very first step is to listen to my body and get off the roids.

Finally, in this moment, I am truly facing the shadow cast on the sidewalk outside Lynn's office after Morfar alerted me to the prison I keep myself in—and deciding to walk away from it.

Just maybe, if I had understood what kind of journey I was about to go on, I would have let truth and balance be.

Truth is always good, but getting there is a bitch.

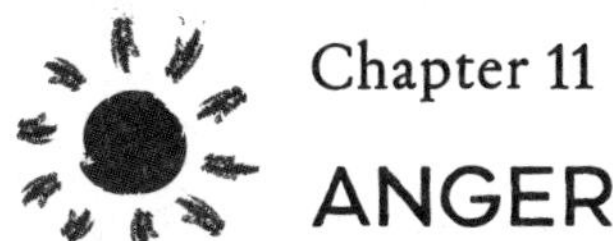

Chapter 11
ANGER

Fuck medicine works at first. The wrath stops hurling, and life turns bearable—until another matter triggers my system into going wayward again.

This time, it isn't medicine but Cal. He calls accusing the babysitter of handling Dandelion inappropriately. His accusations turn out to be a fuss over nothing, but my body doesn't care. A pattern is making itself known: My physical body is displaying my emotional status, the gut being the master indicator. Once a call from Cal or another happening turns it on, my distressed, frenzied gut stays on. Life in our Seaside sanctuary has been a series of loo calls with only a few good intermittences since I went off drugs.

I am once more lying on the pillow, still lime green and wet, this time because of a call from a doctor. My anemia is now so severe that I am daring heart failure if I roll out of bed and into my Jeep to pick up Dandelion from school. But no one else will. In New York, people have lives and jobs and can't cut out to help a friend because there's no social democratic government to hold them up if they're sacked. My friends never say this, but they don't have to. I get it, but I don't get why Cal's answer to my appeal to let Dandelion stay with him while I check into the ER is, "You always fucking want to ruin my afternoon."

Cal has moved on, and I am no longer his go-to. He has a dentist girlfriend with a Wall Street office address, family connections, and her own set of surgical enhancements. So I simply answer, "Fine." I am too depleted from the sack of woes that followed last summer's bad case of food poisoning to get angry.

But I am not fine, and I have to find a way, the MD says—a way to get into the hospital for blood transfusions.

Somehow dark-haired Foster—slender, with proud, hawk-like features and elegant designer clothes that accompany a past in NYC fashion—jumps to mind. He is from around the corner, from one of the estate towns bordering Seaside where known psychologists, like his father, raise their families with piano-playing, pill-popping mothers. But Foster has long traveled the world, at first to find his own medicine, and now to share it. Coincidentally, I had the opportunity to attend one of his workshops months ago.

Being that *Fuck medicine* hasn't cured my ills, I've been looking in other places to right myself. I've browsed and bought stones and sticks, you-can-heal-your-life books, and tarot cards from the shelves at the metaphysical store near Lynn Leclere's office. After a few visits, I realized that Foster couldn't be found at the store, even if a flyer bearing his name could be, and that his Native American Earth-revering way was my way.

A one-day workshop, that's all it took. After all, I am still little Nette, wheeling her hand-me-down red bike as if ripping across the plains like the wind on a magnificent mustang, human and horse together, a tone in the universe, a fullness of existence, unity.

Foster is a shaman, a person with inborn gifts who has apprenticed in native communities and is able to alter his consciousness and enter the unseen world where forces of spirit and nature communicate with him at will. He knows the spirit of the mustang, as he knows other spirits. Unless you've been a visitor to the realm where everything in nature has a voice, a consciousness, you'll think me bonkers for listening to the woman in the store and paying for a workshop with him. Yet I was born with the gift of remembering that we are not separate from Earth—that although we now have Apple for instant connection and science know-how that can manipulate nearly anything, you and I are in the Great Mother's hands, and when we communicate with the creatures whose home we share, life is better, balanced, even beautiful.

Ages of generations in every part of the world have had their own Foster, the priest-healers who have worked for the community with the help of nature. If you ask me today, I'll tell anyone that arrogance has us dismiss this ancient connection. And in dismissing it, we are dismissing ourselves.

Just look at me on the pillow. Look where dismissing my own nature got me. And that's why, months ago, when Foster came to Long Island to reconnect those who needed a shaman to look straight into them with eyes not his own and thumbtack their issues to their awareness so they could finish the job at home, I paid to be one of those people.

Foster offered a space where a room full of successful Long Islanders could be themselves—could connect to something, someone, a nature they had lost. And he did thumbtack my issues, even before I got to join the circle of supporting participants on the mat.

"This girl needs more healing than anyone else in this room," Foster greeted me. He sat cross-legged on the floor, his upper body swaying back and forth while a mystical, wordless song jumped from his throat. "Lie down," he said, barely halting his guttural cadence to get the words out, and patted the mat.

I did, blood rushing to my face and clearing the sapped white of anemia. I had no idea what to expect from the mat or this man, who was the same age as Cal. Within seconds of entering the workshop room, however, I knew I was right where I wanted to be: among strangers and with a man who, in time, would become my spiritual parent. His ability to stream tenderness to strangers while dipping into the cesspool of their lives, pulling out the ugliest pieces to accept, and rearranging their woes for healing with song and energies unseen was like a round yellow moon on a night sky: striking and inviting and, above all, an illumination to see you through.

But then and there, I wasn't entreating spirituality or parenting. I was just hoping for pointers on how to get back to myself.

"Close your eyes." Foster's agile body pendulated next to me, and his hands moved above my body; yet it was his words I hearkened: "This girl—Nette—is white with anger, though she doesn't know what her injustice is. She doesn't know why she is angry. She doesn't know why she rages like Beelzebub has been let loose in her."

The guttural rhythm—the mystical notes pulsing from his throat—took over, trilling softly, while Foster paused, and we became a room etched in a memory of comfortable quietude.

"Anger is a natural emotion and doesn't have to be abusive or hurtful," he continued. "It's a device we can use to set boundaries, and when children are encouraged to vent their anger, they develop a healthy relationship with it and can easily move through this emotion. But if they are taught to ignore and suppress their anger, it becomes an issue for them in adulthood. Over time, repressed anger becomes rage. And rage can kill or start wars. With others and with yourself. Right, Nette?"

Until this moment, his voice had soothed like a lullaby song, but now its pitch changed, and a stricken screech soared.

"You're afraid of going mad, like your mother. But you won't. You are not your mother! Your body's out of control with anger, with repressed rage. And you can't digest the life you chose." The screechiness left as suddenly as it arrived, and Foster's voice shifted to sweet and pleasing again. "That's why you are suffering. And you're dreaming up all these psychosomatic illnesses, each day a new one. Your body and I have already had many conversations about this. It wants to help you, and that's why it has brought you here. We got to get you aligned so you can get in touch with your anger, get in touch with living, and demand to be healthy. And actually live your destiny. Do you understand?"

It's been a while since I left the mat and the room of strangers turned kin, but Foster's words remain a rustle in my ears. Especially now, curled up in the warm comfort of my bed, I cling to his wisdom.

An afternoon of tears was my response when Foster dug into my cesspool and pulled out reasons for my soul-unhappiness. They were tears of relief—relief that I was not going mad, and that my terrible way of being a mother had origins other than being a terrible person. This understanding has lifted one heaviness away from our Seaside home. The workshop hasn't cured me, but the dark-haired shaman has given me a tube of something soothing, something with the power to fix me, if I only follow his directions and apply it.

Deep-seated convictions take time to transform in slow learners like myself, and months had to pass before the shaman's words sunk into my full awareness. In a few minutes, in a room full of supportive strangers, Foster uprooted beliefs occupying a greedy corner in the cloth of my consciousness. He affirmed that I have reasons to be angry, which has taken some getting used to. And who'd know—anger isn't even a bad thing, just a healthy expression, if it moves through you like a smile crossing your lips.

Foster hasn't just been apprenticed in native communities but also at many a family dinner, hosted by a known psychologist, his father, and attended by people like the illustrious psychologist Maslow, and I had never doubted this new truth that he offered me. I get it. Yet if it weren't for the roid rages, I wouldn't even know that some serious anger has settled into me—because what reasons, aside from a few trifles, do I have to be angry? In the big picture of the world, life in the north as a Nilsson has favored me. I come from a good family, raised in one of the globe's rare corners of paradise, absent of otherwise universal hardships like war, dictatorship, and poverty, where space is ample, and nature is a loving—albeit wet and windy—ally, streetlights always work, and a community of neighborly taxes pay your way if bad luck gets you. *What right do I have to be angry?* As Magnum likes to say, I could be cotton-picking somewhere with no shoes, no teeth, and no family.

In this moment, of course, a little hardship has hold of me. I am used up, out of will and words, can't even muster a hiss at Cal, and the MD specialist has me scared enough to know the anemia must improve. *Who will take care of Dandelion if my heart fails? Her dad won't.*

In a striking divorce scene at the mansion, amid dividing up the things we'd carried in moving boxes across ocean and states, Cal's voice had lowered to a rare volume as he whispered across a closed box that it would be best for Dandelion never to live with him. His unhealthy ways would harm her, he said. And we both knew he was right.

Right then and there, I knew our story had ended. And right now, I also know I won't have a blood transfusion. No matter how life-threatening this anemia, I simply won't. I need no more diseases.

I uncurl from the duvet as the MD-sponsored panic retreats. In this, I have an option: There's no better time than now to apply my own tube of medicine, and that's why I'll forgo the blood transfusion and select the alternative the MD doesn't want me to pick. I am going to show her, show this specialist, that it can be done—and while I am doing it, I'll get in touch with my anger.

I am going on bed rest to find my anger and fix my blood.

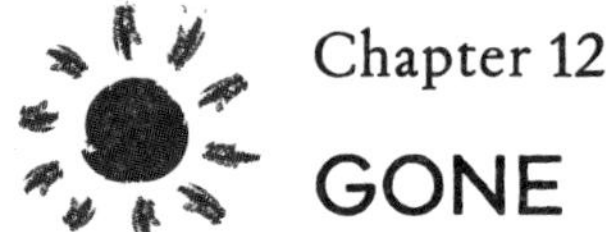

Chapter 12

GONE

There's no telling how long it will take to better the breathlessness that makes a set of stairs seem like a marathon for a bad runner. The MD says any improvement is highly unlikely. Still, I manage to patch together enough sitters for several weeks of almost complete bed rest. I share breakfast and bed with Dandelion and leave everything in between to paid help. And I swallow the new cocktail of drugs the doctor provided; that's the price for avoiding blood transfusions.

I sleep for days, weeks.

But this morning, when I am stirred by the summer sun, which is filtered through tree branches outside the window and streaming into my bedroom in warm patches, I stretch away from sleep and know I am no longer too depleted for words. For the stairs, yes, but not for a yellow pad and a pen that wants to scribble a life of incognito anger away. In that workshop with Foster, he pulled another dark issue from my cesspool, and I haven't forgotten it. There's one more pattern that I want to—*need to*—eclipse, now that he's aired it. There's one other aspect I must bring change upon. The past I inherited, but it's my responsibility to change a familial habit that hurts.

Foster nailed it: I am on track to become a mother who guilts her teenager into staying at home Friday nights because she's all alone and pity-partying after years of husbandless Fridays. The screaming, ugly thing, dripping with resistance, hurt, and injustices when pulled from my dark, is someone who blames others for not doing more, for not relieving the reality my choices have built. There was little lullaby in Foster's tone when he ordered me to stop being a victim, own my power, and follow my dreams. I don't know exactly what that means, but my pen is going to find out. Because I know he is right, again.

Outside, the scorching street is quiet. Only an occasional bee or bird buzzes by. People are at the beach, the pool, or their summer retreat out East. And the hot, lazy silence is like horse dung for the weeds I am about to yank from inside. When your own voice is but a faint murmur, silence is an amplifier, adding power to your soul sound. Silence, therefore, is my new buddy.

I begin by setting the ball of a blue pen against yellow sheets, determined to get in touch with the pieces I have stuffed away.

A page for each name and trust in my pen—that's how I start. Jumping to the first heading, I see the names of Mother Karin and Magnum, and the will of my pen has me scribble below: *Haven't they set me up? For Cal?* I made him a choice in my blueprint, but now a momentous jolt of insight has me sit up in bed way past the sun patches leaving the floor. Am I not merely repeating their stuff? Repeating the familiar? How many times have I heard the story—though Magnum is our storyteller, it's Mother Karin who always narrates this record—of how Nils was blindsided by the elegance of young Karin? Much in the same way I was magnetized by the crisp look of the handsome Ralph Lauren–starring American? And both were mistakes that couldn't be undone, that couldn't be left, because divorce would be dishonorable—a subtle belief passed on from who-knows-where, our inexplicable ancestral baggage.

I remember a few years back, in a windswept moment by Halfdansvej 9's outdoor clothesline, when I joined Magnum as he took a smoke. His chronic jolliness had fled, and tears pressed new frankness to jumble out of him: "I have to divorce her. I can't . . . I can't bear her demands any longer. I can bear her no more."

Mother Karin had started breaking the unspoken rule never to scream or rage when Magnum was home. The black suitcase barely arrived in the hallway before she let out a sound that reached beyond the neighborhood. How fed up she was, having spent thirty years waiting for him and that he'd better retire soon and make up for his awayness. Give her the life she deserved.

Even though I seconded my dad's decision to leave, the frankness never got past the clothesline; Magnum stuck his wife out, couldn't divorce her though he wanted to. And I, too, would have stuck out my mistake if my body hadn't intervened. We are clothesline people, Magnum and I.

Because isn't abandonment owning me, just as it does Mother Karin? The pen moves to remember the upstairs kitchen, so tight that Father Nils had to pull a chair into the doorway from the living room to sit with his coffee while talking to his potato-peeling wife. He was home. The kitchen window fogged up with the warmth of his coffee while I jumped into his lap to help him stir the sugar and sink into his wide, familiar comfort. Then he was gone. A day or two, maybe longer—a three-year-old knows not time—but she did know her dad was gone, not just gone-to-work gone but gone for what seemed like good.

That was an abrupt change, like a punctured tire on a tricycle that stopped all playtime. But she didn't know why—no one told her why the chair stayed in the living room, no one told her Father Nils now worked around the world and she'd better get used to *gone*. Only the way potato peels flew around the kitchen at dinner-prep time told her something.

Her dad returned, but something had changed. The potato peels never landed in the sink again but kept whirling around Mother Karin, even though Father Nils briefly blocked the doorway with the chair, his wide presence, and a new black suitcase. And then he was gone again. And from then on, he showed up only to be gone.

Three-year-old Nette didn't have a name for what settled in her in her father's absence. But I do now. I experienced abandonment, having the parental pillar of comfort upstairs desert me, and that experience marked three-year-old Nette and the person she became.

The pen insists that abandonment is part of the setup for Cal. A hidden part of me fears abandonment, fears being deserted again, fears it like only a big fear can do—non-rational, unexplainable, intrusive—and that's why I couldn't leave. Because I'd rather stick out a marriage mistake, a husband who had two guns and on drunken days made promises to shoot people like Tim McVeigh did, his family included, because they were motherfuckers and shouldn't be in his way, than feel once more what Nette felt the day her dad was gone. Because Cal wouldn't leave me, he would never be gone. He had a good thing, and he knew it. That was a rock-solid, safe bet.

So yeah, I am a different version of Mother Karin, who's been sitting alone at the kitchen table—mornings, dinners, summer evenings—for three decades, waiting, marking time, accepting abandonment. Or perhaps sticking out her own mistake.

In a few honest strokes, the pen strikes down something else, an illusion I've been living with for a lifetime: my happy childhood. In truth, it never was. I didn't have a happy, privileged upbringing like the appearance of our family life would have us and the neighbors think. We weren't a family who had so much; rather, we were a cover story for something that was far from happy, far from balanced, far from healthy. Our story had me fooled. Until now.

That's what cover stories do. They fool.

Indeed, this insight has me speechless, but a moment later the revelation also has me track like a hound, following the trail of blood-truth. I want more. I can't stop.

Truth reveals the wounds that got me sick. Truth heals—if you let it. Which is why another question leaps up from the trail: When did the disease start? When was the point in time I turned away from myself?

Perhaps it wasn't when I got cool at my crossroads moment or with Calvin, but way before. Maybe disease rooted itself when the big blemish roamed the rooms at Friggsvej at leisure, as we are a family who pretends not to see and know the big bad being in the living room, an entity so massive its mere presence squeezes all other activity to a dreamlike slow motion. We deny its existence, or the bad being will have us know we are a family who abandons and who covers it up. Denying what is and living by what looks best, that's the nature of our cover story. That's my family's way, the pen says.

Being six years old is a precious time. Childhood blossoms, and it's the time of Emil from Lonneberga and a wild-haired girl in a yellow sundress, both of whom wake up each dawn to befriend the world and its mysteries. They're fair-haired virgins, a boy and a girl from the north who haven't yet learned all those things we wish children would never discover, and that's outright precious. Emil stays our forever six-year-old, but maybe young Nette slipped away those evenings after dinner when Mormor and she sat at the mahogany table with a blue envelope and a pad of writing paper. Maybe the sundressed girl lost her way then.

From my bed rest silence, I recall watching Mormor calligraphy careful letters onto a white sheet and feeling her sorrow even before she started. Each letter was a careful stroke, a holder for the unspoken tenderness Mormor's upbringing wouldn't have her express. Much later in life, she told me, on one of our coffee dates by the mahogany table when I was on break from UFT, that she wished she were more affectionate, the kind that kissed and hugged and threw I-love-yous to the wind like Grandma Nilsson. But she wasn't. And yet her pen grazed the paper with the same benevolence that had her marigolds dance in brilliant yellows and oranges.

With a six-year-old's forthright acceptance, I whispered, "Conrad and Tobias?" Pause. "Are you writing Conrad and Tobias?"

I was uttering the names I'd been ordered never *ever* to repeat again by Mother Karin's raised index finger, scarily knitted brow, and bent mouth. Only on those evenings, seated at the downstairs table with Mormor as she penned another letter, did I dare whisper the names that oh-so-yearned to steal across my lips. I spoke my cousins' names for us both. Writing them just wasn't enough.

And I heard Mormor, in a tone filled with life's grandest feeling, outdo Grandma Nilsson in affection as she answered, "Yes, I am writing Conrad and Tobias a letter."

In that beat, I knew to coax Mormor into disobeying orders and telling familiar stories about her first-born grandchild and his little brother, near my age, whose absence had her break family rules and pen illicit letters. I knew the stories as well as Mormor did. I remembered my cousins, too, because they played like boys do best. The fruit trees in the orchard at Friggsvej 6 had sheltered not a few of our games in times when all of us, a great big gathering of aunts, uncles, cousins, and parents of different sorts, filled the downstairs for one of Mormor's family events. Until the day when the same unexplained suddenness that took Father Nils away had Conrad and Tobias disappear and be gone for good. And forever after, the rest of the family never uttered their names, ignoring the two lost sons who once were our kin.

One winter evening, the stories ended. Mormor didn't fetch the writing pad from the secretariat. "They never answer my letters anymore." Pause. "And they have changed their last name."

Sometimes, grief fills you with the absence of tears, with not yelling like a mother gone off. Mormor had done all she knew how to so as not to give up on the sons of her son while still respecting her eldest's decision. Through many penned letters, she had let Conrad and Tobias know their seats at the big table would never be removed, even if they had been. In the even-keeled tone of the north, she had let them know they mattered. But this evening, if we had known tears, Mormor would have freed her sorrow onto the table that forever would be short of two boys. My blue-eyed, dark-skinned cousins' name change from Sørensen to their adopted father's name was a hurt that couldn't be mended. Their mother was marrying another man, and their father, Uncle Frank, was forfeiting them as if they were mere chattel. Now, they truly were not our kin.

To this day, I wonder where they are and how they are.

And to this day, Uncle Frank's choice rides him like a mare; without the apples of your eyes, you can never be a seeing man. Yet Frank has never acknowledged the big blemish he and our family created. He has steered clear of it at all times, and Mother Karin has stepped in, raised brows and all, any time conversation has gotten dangerously close to someone naming the unnamable.

Even the neighbors knew not to speak of Conrad and Tobias back then. Young Nette, with a question for everything, was the only trouble. Because it was outright confusing to be told to close your eyes and ask no questions about the big thing in the living room that you didn't understand. That you wanted to understand.

But the adults didn't understand it either. They didn't understand that shame had gotten them to deny two boys of their own, to feign that my cousins never were. In the living room from then on, there was only room for the false story. And young Nette, who counted on Mormor and Morfar for everything—from rye bread dinners to trips to the woods to freshly ironed white linens—could also count on them to forsake, even if they didn't mean to. Perhaps that was the moment when the world lost some of its mystery and disease burrowed in a wild-haired girl in a yellow sundress. I was part of a family where awful truth wasn't allowed. It's what I know.

But the little girl in the yellow sundress deserves to be relieved of living a false story. She deserves to forge her own real version—no blemish, no cover, no danger. That's why I continue on the trail, asking more questions: How come Mother Karin is the ultimate enforcer of our false story? How come she rescued the unnamable from being spoken with the fierceness of Navy SEALS on a mission? *Why is truth so dangerous to Mother Karin?*

I already know the answer, but now I unbind it and let it fall into its place in our story. One shame, two shames, almost the same thing. It happens that Mother Karin is the enforcer of another big, roaming blemish that too long has been blanked out in our family; indeed, some events never occurred, if you ask a Sørensen. She wasn't born this way, knitted brows and going off—at least, not altogether. But if your grandfather starts stroking you when you are a wee lassie, not where most grandfathers would stroke you but in sensitive and private places reserved for later love, this violation blights your sense of self, and you may scream. You may scream so loud and so hard that you get locked up. But if you don't scream, the blight might tear your insides until you can't feel any pain, only numbness. Screams are the only pieces of honesty let out of the story. The rest is trapped inside a big thing you deny, and you will lash out at anyone who dares to point to it. You will become the Navy SEAL on a mission to keep your secret safe.

That's what I think. In reality, I know nothing. I know only what the clues strewn about my childhood tell me. Like Mother Karin, I am endowed with a gift of big intuition, and I intuit that the girl who became my mother had one big blemish that no one would help her dismantle. And then my family's ability to allow trauma to slide into the background set me up for keeping my very own big blemish secret. That's the awful truth.

The pen blurts out that big blemishes are also familiar beings in the Flannery household. New Jersey State Troopers storming the house for a cocaine bust involving two sons on drugs, not to mention the too-friendly priests, all belong in big beings who don't exist at this address. They are too dangerous to have a life. Which is why Cal is familiar with maintaining big blemishes, and why it is little wonder that the awful lie about Kenny grew from a moment before Calvin and I knew each other's names.

The familiarity of a big blemish—that was our true beginning. In the BMW, after spiked rush had torn my back and the American had yelled I was a fucking bitch, out of nowhere a lust of sorts had me bent on cutting the American to pieces the way my posterior just had been. Speaking to his lips, white with bad mood, I told him Black men knew how to dance, unlike white men, who couldn't find any rhythm in their bodies when music wanted them.

This statement sprang forth like a jack-in-the-box jolt, and it got me, and it got him. My sudden assertion had to be another inherited belief, a universal knowingness I drew upon, of a mortal sin, even among Danes then, that Black and white don't screw simply because it makes white men feel bereaved, so much less than the mythical Black penis. The American did react in a big way, and I got to tell him I'd slept with a Black guy, so I knew they knew how to dance.

In this bed rest moment, I remember only that awful word—*cunt*—spewing like a terrible song inside the BMW, and the flaming red of olive skin. The word stung worse than the rush that had cut my back. It was too late to add that the real color of Kenny was sweetness; that he was a soft-spoken UFT student, highly unprepared for the dorm life discrimination a solo Black male student encountered in 1992 in Toronto, and that we first became friends and then one night he brought me to his room and seduced me over talks about basketball. There was no dance, no beat, and no mythical Black penis. We were both outsiders of sorts but not, it turned out, lover material. Soon, Kenny was gone. He went home to his white mama and Black girlfriend, and he gave up his dream of becoming a cop.

That was the God's honest truth about Kenny, but only I knew it. On my first trip to New York, I told Calvin I'd never slept with Kenny—that it all was an awful lie. And that's how our dating started: with a big blemish, as my fiancé wouldn't have a girlfriend who had fucked a Black man. So I hadn't. That was an easy cover-up.

Except this big blemish wouldn't disappear. It takes extraordinary strength and maneuvers to deny the real facts when you're flying high, and it only took a few coke nights for Calvin to interrupt the sensation of greatness with a mission for truth. He wouldn't let the awful lie be, the way we both were used to.

Lying was never my way, just as covers on stories aren't my way, and for one outstanding time I listened to my way. I came clean. And we did fall apart. But we got back together, eventually, and that was a remarkable volte-face. We had named a big blemish, and it almost left our lives. I don't know that anyone in either of our family lines had done this before.

But the shame-whipping didn't leave. It stayed. The awful lie about Kenny gave me a new thing to keep, to endure. The girl who knew sex is a soul connection, sacred, became a whore in her partner's eyes, and I began judging myself for something that was unjudgable to begin with. Not that I caught on. The pen tells me that instead of gaining from naming the big blemish, I lost a big piece of myself in the new shame. That's my family's way—to blank out relationships, events, yourself, so the world will love you back. That's what I knew. Until now.

Just as Calvin was an inevitable choice—a setup, perhaps—Kenny was, too. Mother Karin never ventured downstairs on Friggsvej to join in the TV watching on the state channel, but one evening she appeared in the living room just as a rare sight filled the small screen, as uncommon as that of a singular Black person walking Frederikshavn's downtown streets on an ordinary afternoon. From the screen, The Supremes, with Diana Ross and her big black hair and big colors, sprang out at us alongside big tones of music. Mother Karin moved from the doorway to a seat on the couch next to where I was hidden in Morfar's arm crook. I still hear her words—"Oh, look at her!" And I still feel the zest that moved all of her body as she stayed and watched a strange trio of women sing strange music to a family of four from the north. "Isn't she beautiful? Isn't she ravishing?" She exclaimed her adoration as if she were standing before the West Coast ocean's crashing wildness. Mother Karin has a way of moving others with her screaming and with her glee, because both are unparalleled. Perhaps that moment made my fall for Kenny inevitable, because Black was beautiful in my mother's world.

Aside from big blemishes, there's more to our family story, if you read my yellow pages. Since our move to Halfdansvej

9 we've been the kind of reliable, hardworking, successful steadiness Frederikshavn relies on: Mother Karin, a school board member and Girl Scout leader, and Magnum, an explorer who put our little town on the map as an ambassador for the north, with three kids who were many a teacher's favorite. We've always checked off the right markers for what neighbors gauge an upstanding family to be. Of course, the biggest gauge of all is that we look good, and we look happy. Yet now, from this blue ink, I learn that it wasn't just truth that wasn't permitted growing up—neither were needs.

No needs allowed. That was the barter my parents made for us looking good and happy. So, when Mother Karin was your mother and she had to have some old bricks turned into the equivalent of a spanking-new single-family home while the stringent seventies barely had left, you didn't object when she told you, a mere nine-year-old, that you and your sister had to start pitching in—you had to start working—to pay for the things she wanted you to have.

Mother Karin secured a newspaper job for Sister Sallie and me, despite governmental rules against child labor—one rule she was willing to overlook. In doing so, she robbed me of childhood's final blossom, because I hated each day that I had to bike up a merciless hill, kilos of newspapers on the small frame of a junior bike, against northern chill and darkness, relying only on small wheels and Viking stamina to bring me to junkie town. There, I delivered local news to doors that sprang open with crazed, unclothed men or women who assaulted the paper boy.

Days when Sister Sallie delivered, I hated waiting for my turn the next day. Yet, more than anything in the world, I wanted to ward off the stern look in Magnum's hazy eyes when I pouted. His visits were too short and stern looks were thieves, and he, too, insisted on the junkie town paper route. Objecting or complaining wasn't an option.

I did get a little extra in this barter I didn't ask for and couldn't object to: I got to build character. The Viking stamina is a genetic code, carried to Frederikshavn by the likes of Lars and Anna Emilia, who had to toil and endure as bottom-rung immigrants to survive and give life to more Nilssons, and this part of me jumped to my rescue. I got to know its character. I got to fight my way up a merciless hill, over and over, when that was the last thing I ever wanted to do. Something in me grew wide and deep and indomitable, and it wasn't loathing alone. Wasn't this when the sparkle of six-year-old Nette died and anger—hate, even—began growing roots?

This family way of caring how we looked and not how we felt has no excuse, and I am suddenly angry. I want to hurt Mother Karin. I want to pummel her with my long-standing anger-hurt—but I have no one to beat but a downy bed.

The pen rages across the pages. I am oh-so-very angry about three young kids in their young blossoming who got robbed. When you are nine and twelve and you live in a rare corner of paradise, it is your job to play and goof off and run with boys, not have an overshadowing job to help pay to look better than the neighbors. Sooner or later this kind of work not only supersedes your needs but also leaves you with no needs, which is absolutely against human nature, so you try to fill the needs of others to feel something—for example, those of an American with a drug habit and a bag of woes.

In the hours that follow, the pen takes all of it to the pages—the unfairness, the injustice, the anger at Mother Karin. Sheet upon sheet upon sheet, until I fall asleep.

WHEN I AWAKE, the angry roar of my pen takes a sudden hit at Magnum, even if he was always a challenge to be angry with, as he never failed to kiss you goodnight, and in the north, where showing affection was like a French verb everyone dodged, his hugs were unparalleled. But my pen has no trouble today. Anger shoots across the sheet because of the Royal Caribbean Cruise ad Magnum insisted we imitate: a mock display of father, mother, brother, and sisters Nilsson on a giant white ship gliding across the wide ocean in glimmering sunset, beautiful ladies wearing gowns and gems waltzing with gentlemen in tuxedos to flowing one-two-three counts of Johan Strauss while children sit on seats with big smiles, just watching—altogether a content picture of peace and happiness, of familial success. The ad for the Royal Caribbean Cruise was Magnum's ideal family, and he demanded that we jump on the white ship and play along. Every one of us. Every visit home. A stern look in his hazy eyes, or a rare smack of a big hand against the wayward, had us comply.

He, of all people, ought to have known a child needs not a job but needs themselves. Yet in the end, however difficult it is for me to take on board, Magnum has always cared more about us looking happy than he has about our needs being met. He and Mother Karin agree on something: Halfdansvej 9 has always been a joint deal.

Between the rounds of yellow pages, new exhaustion gets me, and I lose time to sleep again. Changing the picture of my childhood, of myself, and of those around me, is arduous work.

WHEN I AWAKE, the Magnum worship on Friday nights beckons. These nights, we gathered around the TV like a family antsy with anticipation before the opening of a big circus performance. Watching Magnum made us feel right. We adored a man on the screen, the man the world saw, and we looked good and happy doing so. Still, despite the growing coffers, the price of awayness to pay for good and happy, of connecting with a TV signal but not the real Magnum, added to the things stashed away. The price of awayness is dear. The price of love is dear. That's what I know now.

Next, in a striking moment, glee gets me. Sheets, lime green, exhaustion, blue-colored writing—no matter, glee takes hold of my drained body and makes every cell jump in exuberance as if Diana Ross or the wild ocean has appeared. Because I *get* what my body has been trying to tell me all this time. I need to be happy. My way, the soul-happy way. I now see where happy never was, where it was misdirected like a malfunctioning signal that points you in the wrong direction. The better we looked, the worse we felt, in the north and in my marriage.

This bombshell epiphany is outright a jubilant rest stop on the trail, and I submerge myself in the joy of finally making sense of where the desire for soul-happiness was conceived. Soul-happiness is the six-year-old's way, and I need to make it my way again.

I soon finish the last angry sheet with Magnum's name on top. Another injustice, perhaps, that my pen is much harder on Mother Karin, who never went away and never turned into a TV signal, but who on good days had hot chocolate and *varme boller* ready after school, before the paper route called. That injustice deserves, "I'm sorry."

And I am. Sorry.

Babysitters come and go below while the blue ink catches other matters that have been hidden, obscured, a falsehood, until now about my family. In an abrupt second, all doubt about hate leaves. No *perhapses* or *maybes* pop up. Because I do hate. And no lime green can cool the hatred claiming my hand and all of me. *I hate Mother Karin.* I hate my mother with more than my might. I hate her with a torrent greater than any mad river, greater than any roid rage, greater than the greatest, wildest ocean beating the shore. My dreams were big, boundless, beautiful, and also bold, but they were robbed from me, mercilessly, at a dinner table on an ordinary wintry evening when I was fifteen and didn't anticipate anything but another dinner. The hate that followed was also big, boundless, and bold, but only beautiful in its persistence to endure inside a daughter who didn't even know she hated her own mother so. Because her father told her she mustn't.

On an ordinary late afternoon, daylight long gone, Little Penis sat next to Mother Karin, and Sister Sallie and I squared mother and son at the kitchen table. Knives and forks moved *frikadeller* and potatoes away from the white dinner dishes. Mother Karin led the silence.

Inside my head a good day—a great day, even—roamed. Next to me lay a piece of paper requiring Mother Karin's signature. Trill and thrill connected me to the sheet, invisible promises of what was to come, of what had been inspiring my Canadian stories since I was the woolly-headed kid sitting on stairs waiting for the town bus to drive by and conjuring a future where all was possible. A big roll of yellowness bounced inside me.

"Mrs. Simonsen wants you to sign this," I said. "Parental approval is required for a Gymnasium application." I wanted to tuck the paper away in my school bag, ready for my teacher tomorrow, sooner than soon.

Mother Karin looked at me, away from the silent space her gaze occupied during meals. "What for?"

"I want to attend Gymnasium, to become a journalist." With my inborn yearning for stories and knowledge, I had sucked a lot of people dry over the years—and with the paper next to me, there was no reason not to share my unaired ambition and a bit of my great day. Given my years of slamming on a typewriter, my desired career could hardly be a surprise choice.

"Hahaha! You want to become a journalist! Hahaha." Mother Karin caught Sister Sallie's eyes and another set of cackling joined in, a mean chorus. "She wants to become a journalist, do you hear? Hahaha. Don't you know where you come from? Hahaha. Your father is blue-collar, he uses his hands to make money, he's a nobody, and so are you. You can't do this. You don't have what it takes. You can't become a journalist. Absolutely not!"

How does a fifteen-year-old cope with her world collapsing over a meal of potatoes and *frikadeller*? I was the girl who was going somewhere. Everyone knew so . . . everyone but my own mother.

While Little Penis left the table, I learned Mother Karin wouldn't have my back; she wouldn't have my dreams, but she would have my sister scorn me for the little big thing inside of me that I nourished like Morfar nurtured his Kadet. She would rob her child's dream, and like doing it. She would have me go nowhere.

Nothing could ever have prepared me for this awful dinner table moment where I met a Dream Robber, my mother, who dishonored the life, the power, she had given me. This turn of events was outright inconceivable.

Space stood still until I managed to squeak, "But I need to make a decision about where I am going after public school. And I want to attend Gymnasium."

"You need to attend tenth grade and then Handelsskolen. Where blue-collar belongs. That's it!" Mother Karin announced her verdict, the worst possible alternative, locking the doors on my future with a fresh smile. Silence had left the dinner space.

In my family, we don't bang doors, we don't hang up, we don't yell, and we don't storm away from a dinner table. But on this late afternoon nothing mattered but my need, and I jumped up and fled from Mother Karin and Sister Sallie. I couldn't have them witness the tears in my eyes. I didn't know what to do with all that awfulness, not in their presence.

I am learning now why I have avoided hugging Mother

Karin all those times when I have returned for a visit, why I've avoided calling her unless Magnum is present for backup. Like shame-whipping, hate has stuck.

Later that evening, Magnum happened to call from Czechoslovakia, where his job took him often in the mid-eighties. I settled on the shiny staircase to listen in on the phone conversation drifting from the kitchen. She could rob me of my dream, perhaps, but not my will.

As the Magnum-Karin call was coming to an end, I did another thing we don't do in my family: I swept into the kitchen and—placing myself in front of Mother Karin, who was leaning on the counter with the landline receiver against her ear—reached for the phone, not hiding the steel of my intention. "I want to speak to my father," I demanded in a tone full of pluck and force.

In my family, children do not make demands. If something was not offered or given, it was not for Nette to ask for it, let alone demand it. But on this night I didn't care about family rules. I had to speak to my father, no matter what it took to get him on the line.

My sudden appearance in the kitchen startled Mother Karin. Her face froze, and I grabbed the phone out of her hand. Skipping the obligatory greeting, I sputtered my anguish into the receiver.

"She won't let me attend Gymnasium, and I need a parental signature to get admitted. She says I'm blue-collar and wants me to attend tenth grade and then Handelsskolen. She won't sign the paper." I hurled the words into the receiver to give my father all the facts in case Mother Karin tried grabbing the phone.

Never before had I spoken this bluntly to my father. Never before had I been this vulnerable. "I want to become a journalist and write for a big paper that covers political issues around the globe. That's my dream, but she won't have it.

Tenth grade is optional and Handelsskolen is the wrong track for journalism. It's not at all what I want to do!"

I paused my whirl of words, at last listening for my dad on the other end.

"Of course you can attend Gymnasium. That is a good dream you've got, kiddo. I am proud of you." Magnum's warm, consoling voice reached me past several countries. In an instant, he made everything all right, and I knew my dream was secure. "I will sign the paper when I get home next week."

"Thank you, Dad," I whispered.

Speaking frankly to my father about something that involved Mother Karin—and being met with understanding—was a novel experience. Magnum got my dream, and I was going somewhere again. Expecting that I could be frank about other matters, I added in a normal tone: "I never want to speak to her again. Ever. She makes life miserable, and I can't bear it." Once more, I was doing what we don't do in my family. I was letting Magnum know all that felt not good and happy at home.

His voice was still warm and sonorous when he responded, "Can't you just get along with your sister and mother? Be nice and don't make war with your mother. I just want you all to be happy." A small sigh accompanied his answer.

"Yes," I mumbled, all out of pluck and force. This rare phone call was becoming one of Magnum's postcards—glossy prints of cities, countrysides, and festivals from distant places strewn in an entire childhood, a collection of beautiful pen strokes reminding me to be a good girl and help my mother because she needed it, signed by a father who hoped we all were happy. Despite the sweet reminder of a caring presence away somewhere, the postcard never made young Nette feel very happy. Heading up the hill to junkie town and helping my mother were tied for last thing I ever wanted to do.

But I had to do both and feel good about it, because now

Magnum insisted anew, "*Shhh* and be a good girl," on the phone from Czechoslovakia. He would support any dream, but no emotions that got in the way of being a well-trained and agreeable daughter. Such sentiments were simply not allowed.

I turned to hand Mother Karin the receiver.

Just like being told to keep the peace and make yourself uncomfortable so others can remain comfortable, this was another bad barter young Nette didn't ask for. With the chronic inflow of postcards, I was asked to dishonor my own signaling system, the stop sign that told me what was going on was unacceptable. Except it had to be acceptable. *Be good, look good, and zip up about what's going on* had to be acceptable.

But the unacceptable will express. Give it time, and it will.

Future dreams were also forfeited at the dinner table because the moment before I—a semi-precious fifteen-year-old with a good dream—voiced my innermost wish can never be restored, no matter Magnum's support. Beware. Words of a mother are powerful, and they can rob absolute faith in dream-making. Words like, "You can't do this. You don't have what it takes," uttered with zest and scorn, can settle in you and appear at important junctures like another misbehaving signaling system, mucking up your blueprint.

Foster's deep-throated voice reminds me now that when your mother has a dream, you're halfway there. I never got that halfway, however, because Mother Karin forgot the power of dreaming, forgot the notebook she'd filled with stories rich in her kind of wildness, long before I turned fifteen—and that was a sacrifice, for her and for me. When your dreams are denied, an ominous shadow takes over you and you live your shadow's life, not your life. That's where I am.

Foster's voice reminds me again, like another pen stroke in the bedroom uttering forthrightness, to own my life, to follow my dreams. This advice seems rather simple, now that I see where I lost my dreams.

Even so, the *End* hasn't yet been reached on the yellow sheets. The pen seeks to know why a trail of postcards persisted in reminding me to take care of Mother Karin.

Chores were sensible requests to make of us children to help our household function. Yet wasn't Magnum reminding young Nette to do more than chores? Wasn't he also asking her to reach Uncle Frank to have him come rushing with a bag of medical tricks to knock out a head-banging Mother Karin those times when breakdown got her? There are dots in my childhood, each one feeling like a winter trip to a Siberian outpost in light summer garments—images of Mother Karin with froth around her mouth, banging her head into a wall or some other hard surface, over and over, while screaming her loudest, maddest scream. The pen begs why Magnum thought young Nette and Sallie were prepared to help their mother in this way. Didn't he know time seemed awfully eternal when they stood next to a woman gone mad in the mudroom, attacking a washing machine with her head and the air with her screams, while waiting for the quiet rescuers, Uncle Frank and his syringe, to arrive? Or for their mother to return to the world, which never happened on its own? Their uncle was always somehow magically called, as if an invisible being forced the dial each time a dot appeared.

Frank had gotten into medical school following falling victim to a rare, flesh-eating disease as a teenager. A rotting leg had him hospitalized for a year and disqualified him from the shipyards. Though doctors insisted upon amputation, his mother's balanced way and will saved his limb; she went against doctors, not a small thing in the obedient fifties, and plain refused amputation. She wouldn't have her child crippled. There had to be another way, Mormor maintained.

And there was. Penicillin—a new and untried drug at the time—saved Uncle Frank's leg. And as Mormor had savings from her parents' brewing business, her son got to go to medical school following his bed rest year. Aging nurses in Frederikshavn still remember "Beautiful Frank," who had an easy way and his own brand of zest before life hardened him. He doctored innumerable cases of people at their lowest and craziest and knew what to do with the least intervention possible—including for his own sister—and he pulled Mother Karin away from the edge and into bed each time.

Every head-banging dot shared a common flow: a desperate situation, Frank sweeping in, nothing spoken, injection, Frank sweeping out, leaving two young girls and a small boy at a loss for how to name the awful happening. The next dawn, Mother Karin jumped out of bed, like she did on any other day, and the dot stayed nameless, covered. Perhaps that's what Magnum intended with his caring postcards to me and to my sister. But this kind of help—protect your mother so she doesn't hurt herself, but do shush and cover it up—is a big favor to ask. It's asking for no truth, no need, and no emotion all in one go.

My real childhood did, in all ways, set me up for Cal—set me up for stuck and soul-unhappy.

And now, as Morfar entreated, the unhesitating pen turns to forgiveness: I must let myself off the hook, now. The pen does forgive all the times I stayed, all the times I couldn't leave a mad husband or a husband gone mad. A replica of young Nette holding space for her mother's delirium until help arrived had me stay, had me stuck. Yet the hardest dot for the pen to find clemency for is one that appeared well past childhood: Cal arrived in the mansion kitchen and his black bag landed on the stone floor with a hollow thud. His eyes were bloodshot, and not because he'd taken a red-eye flight from Las Vegas—or perhaps exactly for that reason. A new deal with a big client had just been bagged in a casino, in a lit-up glitzy hotel, or maybe over a lineup of lines.

Dandelion crawled over to greet her dad while I finished rinsing something at the sink.

"What fucking way is this to greet the king?" Cal paid no attention to the little figure clutching his pants; he looked straight at me. "Where are the servants? Why aren't they lined up to greet me? They should be outside in the driveway when I make my entry. I *am* the fucking king! What have you done to them? What?"

At the sink, I noticed my hands stiffening, reeling motionless in the air. The bellowing, the anger was standard. That was my husband's way. But the rest was new. I needn't look at Cal to know this was no crack-a-joke attempt. Behind me, I heard him move into the pantry, then the adjoining dining room. "Where are they? Where are you hiding them? Where are the low-life servants? You got them cooking up some poison, because you're all working for the FBI. You fucking cunt. I knew I shouldn't have trusted you."

I grabbed Dandelion, hugged her tightly, and trailed my husband. Even though I'd been trained for times like these during Mother Karin's head-banging episodes in my childhood, the chill was awful. Every part of me turned to ice.

Cal strode up the long oak staircase, but abruptly he stopped and peered into the Tudor ceiling, high above him, whispering and mumbling. That was also new. Cal had never been one to whisper.

Sudden sadness pushed away the Siberian chill inside me. Standing at the bottom of the stairs, I spoke softness, a plea of its own. "You need help, Cal." This was more than common paranoia. "You are hearing voices. You need help. Please!"

"You fucking cunt." He looked away from the ceiling. "You better watch out. Tim McVeigh had it right when he took down all those people. I will, too, and if the servants aren't back when I return, I got a Glock to make it right."

Perhaps the hardest thing, the obstacle the pen just can't seem to write by, is my knowing that if I were not hugging a diaper-clad figure in my arms, her chubby flesh brushing mine, her breath a warm reminder of a future, I would have stayed one more time. I would have stayed until the end, until the Glock was aimed at me.

Success, the stress of success, and the white lines that now came with success were a new combo. My husband knew no limits, and the voices spoke against me; they would have no happy ending. Still, I would not have run. That is one huge, enormous unpardonable dot, and if my pen can find mercy for this, it can find mercy for anything.

The self-help books are finally making sense. I do need to love myself, care for *me*, or I will always be the mother who left a potentially deadly situation for her daughter, but not for herself. That is no longer the person I choose to be. My body won't have it. I won't have it. It's unacceptable.

That's how truth liberates, how it sets you free. That's the true healing power of truth.

Outside my bedroom door, a timely ruckus happens. Dandelion is no longer a patient little girl who takes her place next to her mama in the evening with a stack of books she'll read aloud to the bedroom. No longer is she the girl who forfeits needs and emotions—because even before the discoveries on the truth trail, I knew to let Dandelion own her woes.

Now, she lets me know something isn't right in her world; her screams, fits, and floor-hugging outside the bedroom door make clear that she wants to be set free of babysitters. She wants to be a regular four-year-old whose mother isn't locked in a bedroom fortress. Even Kathleen can't hold her spellbound anymore with summer discoveries and ice cream trips. Dandelion wants her mama. Enough is enough.

My little girl is right. Eight weeks is enough. A beloved, truth-seeking pen has set me free of the unknown predators of my past, has helped me garner peace with the childhood that never was, the cover stories and dark spots in and around me. The pen has taken me to the end of the trail, and I am no longer daring heart failure. Bed rest has worked.

In the thousands of pen strokes behind me lie clarity and forgiveness for the people, covers, and shadows we have been and are. The pen found me clemency. Life is making sense, and that's a rejuvenation that can't be bottled, reciped, or even described, because it starts in the blood and ends in the soul.

I throw the downy cover aside and jump out. My girl needs her mother, and I need to show Dandelion the new me.

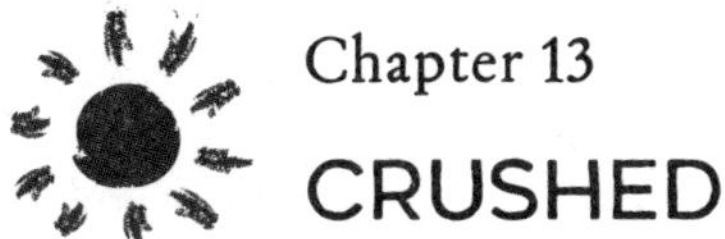

Chapter 13
CRUSHED

Sometimes spry new beginnings are felled by universal nudges. All good intentions and rejuvenation from healing your blood on bed rest are crushed by something much, much bigger than you—something like a formidable thunderstroke, as if Thor himself has aimed all of his will into striking you in a frail spot with no name on a good day in June.

The calendar shows June 13, 2005. Dandelion is buckled into the back of the Jeep. Three generations down our line, she's the only shareholder of Mormor's fine oval face and features, though her loquaciousness isn't from the north. On good days like now, the Cherokee is alive with giggles. Dandelion doesn't require Katthult or Kirseholt to spot quirks in the world and laugh with them.

I am giggling, too, simply because my girl is making me do so, and that's a precious good moment, the kind you return to in the future when you realize how outright blessed you were in that stretch of Jeep time.

Perhaps I don't have all that much to giggle about. Though bed rest is over, and I am out of the danger zone for heart failure, months later my body hasn't yet caught up. Letting go of a false childhood, cover stories, hate, rage, and other stuff needs some adjusting to, and my body isn't yet accepting that a new system has been installed. Imagine the tracks on thirty-some years of signaling. Like those of a well-used train route, they can't be replaced overnight, no matter my wishes or expectations. Woes, old and new, are still with me.

From a point in the future, I understand that gentleness and patience is oft what's most required, not just for our minds but for our bodies as well. They do so much work—underappreciated work. They hold us. They guide us. They move us. They host our souls. They are our main address. That's a lot of work, laborious work, and they don't receive nearly enough appreciation and gentleness. Certainly not from me in this Jeep moment, because even though I am giggling, I am fed up with my body and its ailments. Be patient, be tender with your body; it is another blessing taken as a given. In a future now, I get how it is only a given until it is taken.

The black Jeep rolls down our tree-lined street aburst with vivid dog day colors in a contemporary American version of a good Morten Korch story—that is, a Danish fairy tale–like drama about good and evil set in picturesque settings with a superb happy ending. Just now, goodness reigns in and around my girl and myself in the Jeep. Life is in order. Life is making sense.

On the empty passenger seat, my black Nokia flashes a Florida area code. I yank the vehicle into a vacant spot around the corner and answer the call.

And everything changes.

"Hello," I say. *What does he want now?*

These days the Sea Ray I don't co-own is parked in South Beach, where Cal has taken up residence. Finding good parking spots for his yacht and captaining it up and down the Eastern Seaboard, that's his new occupation. IService hasn't made it far into the new century, despite a solid pipeline of projects.

Cal's apartments in Minnesota and Manhattan have been shut down. Divorcing wasn't good for maintaining timelines.

"Is this Nette Nilsson?" A deep, all-man voice mispronounces my name. The fellow obviously doesn't know me.

"Yes," I confirm.

"My name is Christian Sanchez. I am a detective with the Miami-Dade Police Department."

Oh no! Has he been arrested? Has cocaine finally caught up with Cal? A heavy tug grabs my gut, even if he is ex to me. *Dear God, no!*

Strangers are sometimes those kindest to you. The pause that follows is a thoughtful, caring gesture from the detective who knows some of what he is about to cause.

The sky turns dark, birds stop chirping, flowers die, all brightness leaves, and the world freezes in a forever no one ever would want or hope for. The moment is a Morten Korch apocalypse.

Sanchez's voice is slow—tender, even—when he speaks next. "I am calling about Engelhardt Nils Nilsson."

Stop. Just stop. Stop. Yet the roar of grief won't listen. It is unstoppable, voiceless, soundless; it starts like thunder in the chest and explodes inside my body and takes everything along. I am pain. The world is pain. Sanchez need not say what comes next. Grief and I already know that the unfathomable, what just can't be, is.

Although the roar of grief is powered to shake all of Mother Earth, I only let out a singular sob—"Please no!" My chest is gone, my body is gone, annihilated by the ungraspable that never was written into our story. Not him. Not Magnum. Not my dad. *No! No! No!* Not my dad. It's all too soon.

"We have attempted to call Karin Nilsson but could not reach her. Are you Mr. Nilsson's daughter?"

"Yes, I am . . . Is he . . . is he?"

"Yes, Ms. Nilsson, I am very sorry to report that your father was found deceased in a Marriott Courtyard hotel room in

Miami early this afternoon by a maid—at 2:40 p.m., to be exact. I am so sorry for your loss."

No amount of kindness and caring in the voice of a manly Miami-Dade detective can change the time tick when true darkness arrives and seizes everything. The indelible "no more" happens so swiftly. My dad is gone. Really gone. Really gone for good. Big, brawny, jolly Magnum. The pillar and strength of our family, the optimist, the forgiver, the giver, he who always saw the best in others. No more.

Overwhelming devastation takes over the Jeep.

"An autopsy is scheduled to determine the principal cause of death, but it appears that he died from natural causes—atherosclerotic heart disease. There is some trauma to his neck; he must have hit the nightstand on his way down."

"Did he suffer?" I whisper. That is what I need to know.

"I don't believe so," Detective Sanchez responds. "The autopsy report will give more detail, but I believe it was instantaneous." Pause. "It seems he'd just returned to the hotel room and was getting ready for bed. He was wearing undergarments only. White ones."

Damn the new clients. Damn Florida. Damn the call that should have been about Cal, not my dad. Damn it all.

And then I cry. I cry while Detective Sanchez listens. He seems in no rush to finish this awful call.

When the cries cease, he shares a few last details: "Your father didn't show up for a scheduled breakfast at a client site, and after several hours had passed, the client made a call to his hotel, the Courtyard on Seventy-Seventh Street in Miami Lakes. Apparently, they believed it was out of character for your father not to show, and a maid was sent to the room to check on Mr. Nilsson. Ms. Nilsson, I am going to give you my phone number and you can call any time of day or night with questions. The autopsy and police reports will be available on . . ."

After Detective Sanchez leaves the call, I stare at the Nokia and a chortle emerges. A maid! Imagine writing that into your blueprint: I intend to be found by a Hispanic maid in an American hotel, far away from my Danish family, wearing white underwear. This scenario is our family way, and I laugh because it *is* funny, and because I don't have enough body to let out the grief that I am.

"Mama, what is it?" Dandelion's silver-bell voice reaches me from the back seat. Her giggles have turned quiet.

"Come here, sweet pea." I reach for my girl, and she jumps into my hug. I wrap my arms around her soft preciousness and tell her she can't have a chicken quesadilla tonight because her morfar has gone to heaven.

"Why did he have to go today?" Dandelion mumbles against my skin. Taco Bell is another thing she gets to miss, though today she won't have any fits or do any floor-hugging. She's my daughter, and when times go rough she turns off everything that could make the tumbling of her world worse.

Yes, why now? How could you do this to us, to Mother Karin? Couldn't you have waited, say, a few decades?

Then we smile, because love will have us smile. Magnum has given us infinite reasons to smile and infinite reasons to feel the warmth of our chests and the good mood of our spirits. And that is what we do. We hug and we smile and we love Magnum, who has sprinkled our lives with so much goodness and so many jokes. He had a joke for everything. Even his own departure.

We love him so.

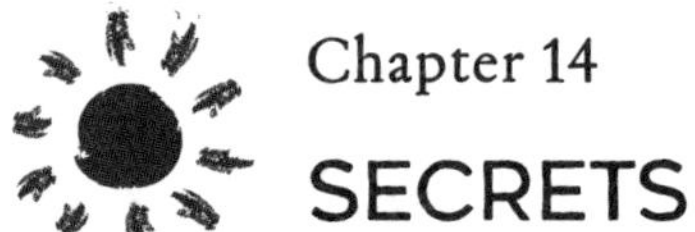

Chapter 14
SECRETS

At the house, I have a call to make, a dreaded call that will shatter someone else's world. In a fortnight, Mother Karin's life—the life she'd been killing time in anticipation of for years, thirty-two years to be exact—was going to begin. She is retiring from her late-life career at the ferry line, and she was going to finally be with her husband full-time, sharing his pad in Atlanta and joining him in various hotel rooms across the US.

Mother Karin does have a dream, after all. Except now that it is time for it, the dream has been killed.

Never for a second do I consider calling Mother Karin. Mother Karin is fragile, and I—we—must protect her. That was the unwritten intent of all those postcards.

I wish to freeze time, to annul the tick before the Florida code flashed on the Nokia and devastation shook my world. But more than anything, I wish for a magic shield so big it will protect Mother Karin and her dream.

I dial my sister's number to share the details of Detective Sanchez's devastating call.

Sister Sallie need not describe the screaming that escapes Halfdansvej 9 after she has stirred Mother Karin out of sleep on a dream-robbing dawn in June. No one has ever met greater grief than Mother Karin in her chair by the kitchen table, lamenting and head-banging her loss onto a designer surface—a gone husband and dream—which no syringe will save her from, despite Sallie calling Uncle Frank for backup. Sallie and I stay in close contact in the hours that follow while Frederikshavn and the world wake up to a Magnum-less place. Sometimes death is a beautiful thing; if only it weren't so damn permanent.

The kitchen at Halfdansvej 9 quickly fills with people and calls from around the town, country, and world—not just family and friends but also acquaintances, work buddies, and clients turned pals—a jumble of relationships carved out of decades of traveling the globe, innumerable voices who all speak their shock and sorrow to the kitchen, in person, on the phone, or in emails and letters. "Suddenly and all too soon," their bafflement says, "an immortal man gone." Without fail, those we know and those we don't know all mention the postcards, the thoughtful postcards, they received for their birthday or a holiday, for years reminding them they were worthy of beautiful pen strokes and a stamp.

On this terrible, dream-robbing day, Little Penis is called next, and in moments he and his wife, Poline, pack up their wagon with two toddlers, leave his banking career in Luxembourg, and head home to join in grief. Brother and sisters, our families, and Mother Karin . . . each one of us must be recalling last Christmas Eve, when we were gathered at Halfdansvej 9 for another wonderful setting—nay, a magical one.

Magnum was, as always, our centerpiece; good humor and feel-good set in quite naturally when he was home, especially on this particular Christmas Eve, as every one of us was there. The Morten Korch god had arranged for a fine layer of snowflakes to fall on the world outside like sweet, soft music notes dancing down. Magnum's favorite album—Bing Crosby's classic carols, played every Christmas since the album was bought in the seventies—was spinning on repeat. The kids played gaily; there were no strained voices. Mother Karin outdid the duck and gravy, and later we sang the psalms and walked around the Christmas tree, as tradition has it, adding that extra touch of magic to a family finally gathered in unison and in peace.

It was an exceptional Eve, and perhaps Magnum knew, *I finally did it. They are all happy.*

We were.

And I can leave.

That's what my intuition says, across the Atlantic on the soil I still share with my dead dad.

Sometimes it is your child who is kindest to you. Even if she is a mere five-year-old, or perhaps for that exact reason, kindness makes Dandelion go through her library of photos, boxes of them, and pick out visual memories of Morfar Magnum. "They're for you," my child says, extending her stack of kindness. "So you won't be sad," she adds.

I behold a handsome, tanned Magnum sitting with a large draft in his big hand. He's at an outdoor café with Mother Karin and two-year-old Dandelion one summer when we visited a neighboring town to enjoy fresh-caught seafood.

Maybe my little girl also recalls last summer, when, just before bed rest began, she and I flew to Atlanta to spend Memorial Day weekend with Magnum. An endless sequence of clients, flights, and drives across America had never before given way to a break in Magnum's schedule to have us visit, not until this extended weekend in his new Peachtree apartment located in the same complex as the former, smaller pad with no office. Rain canceled our plans, and we spent the weekend in the apartment, where comforters, corners, and counters had all been scrubbed for our arrival. Morfar and Dandelion took a trip to CVS and returned with more Polly Pockets than one store possibly could house. They settled in Magnum's office, from which a trail of questions, patient answers, and chatter made it to the bedroom I occupied. Magnum and Dandelion alone—no other relative interfering—was a first, and proved a combo that produced drawn drawers, rummaging, and giddy laughter. I didn't know what Magnum was showing and telling Dandelion, or she him, but morfar and grandchild found each other that rainy weekend in Atlanta.

The rain was all too short, and we had to leave this exclusive, one-of-a-kind experience with Magnum.

The following morning, he called me. He missed us, he said. The apartment was empty without us two kiddos.

Magnum hugs and kisses and helps you, but he never tells you he misses you—that's bad for business.

I told him I missed him, too.

Silence. Not a pause, but silence.

And then: "I love you. You know that, don't you? *Jeg elsker dig.*"

I didn't know how to react, not to this version of Magnum and to the fact that I was thirty-four years old and for the first time in my life hearing my dad tell me he loved me.

No matter what, I am a truth-seeker, and when Mother Karin, all out of screaming, consents to speak to me, I ask her a question. I can't just let it be. I can't just let the universal nudge be. I have to invite it along. I can't just let Magnum be gone in peace.

The universal nudge responds: *You're a truth-seeker, right. You want to know? Everything, right?*

Truth heals, remember that. But getting there is such a bitch.

Before I unload what's on my mind, Mother Karin tells me about the call from Magnum a mere few hours before his last departure. He'd just returned from the client plant and decided to wake his wife up with a brief chat. "How are you? The midnight shift's running like a dream. I'll call you tomorrow."

I tell her I need to go to Atlanta. I need to go now, before our flight to Denmark in two days.

Mother Karin won't agree. Her answer, in fact, is an outright *No!*—until I remind her about the Green Bay–based family business that recently purchased Magnum's longtime Danish employer. If I don't go, some bureaucrat from Wisconsin is going to pack up everything, from Magnum's shoes to computers. Someone else is going to remove the medley of kiddo photos on his tackboard and count the gin and tonic bottles in the garbage. Magnum shared much with the world, but not his privacy. The last thing I want to do for him is honor the other home he made in Atlanta.

At last, so does Mother Karin. She gives me the go-ahead and bids me to bring home the pink set of golf clubs Magnum bought her, an early retirement gift.

THE NEXT MORNING, I am standing on the burning tar of a modern apartment complex, peach trees abounding on the trimmed grounds, a picturesque setting but for the humidity and the two-bedroom dead zone I am about to enter. I'm in good hands; I know so within seconds of meeting Charles. This middle-aged, pudgy figure, who looks more like someone steering a harvester than an international business, is the new owner and has flown down to assist me in cleaning out Magnum's private items. Sure, he has an interest in ensuring I only remove what is Magnum's, and he may be Green Bay all the way, but he's also a gentleman. His warm eyes, the tears that peek at the corners when he hugs me, and easy company say so.

He unlocks Apartment 212 and tells me to do what I need to do, and call if I need help. We agree on three different piles—one for me, one for Green Bay, and one for the dumpster—and then he takes out a paper and settles in my dad's American armchair.

Atlanta traffic and two return flights await in the late afternoon. I have five hours to complete the mission Charles doesn't know about. How would he or anyone know? I look the farthest from someone doing undercover work, frail and afflicted from much more than sudden grief, struggling with the weight of the black Samsonite suitcase I am about to fill. I am a physical mess, but I have to find answers to the questions that have been with me for a lifetime. No one else will.

Inside the space that just was my dad's, the scent of my childhood hovers. Old Spice and hints of tobacco swirl in an exclusive warmth, Magnum's own brand, the best brand ever, now trickling away. A few more days and my dad's scent will be gone. My chest explodes again, and I almost drop onto the thick blue carpet, hugging it like Dandelion while screaming like Mother Karin. But a mission and two flights that won't wait have me push my shoulders back and still the body's mourning signals. I can't give in—not now, not here, not with Charles in the chair.

I start by walking a slow round to honor the man whose belongings I am about to fleece, to honor his second home. He makes me proud. Everything is washed, cleaned, and put away.

I enter his bedroom, just a standard double bed with a navy comforter, a large mass-produced framed print hanging above it, two nightstands, and a closet.

As I slide the closet door open, my chest does it again. Grief wants out, but that's an explosion I can't let happen. This is so hard. Every touch and glance I ache to have last past the tick of time. I focus on hangers lined up, clothes folded in stacks on shelves, shoes in a precise row below. I reach for my dad's coat, the one that Mother Karin has begged him to discard for years, and I don't ever want to tear myself from something that smells so wonderfully, thickly, of my father. I give myself time to fill nostrils and chest with the last bit of him before I go looking for the answers, before he disappears.

They are here, somewhere. Aside from the clothes, this is a soulless bedroom; the only foible are stacks of wrapped Fruit of the Loom underwear belonging to someone who fears a shortage.

I won't find the truth here. I grab some things for my pile and move on.

I speed toward the kitchen. Cabinets are stocked with common dishes and unwanted knickknacks once belonging to Nanghsi, and an unexpected assembly of spices. The dumpster pile quickly grows. *Forgive me!* Before the fridge door, everything stills. Here hangs Magnum's most prized possession: fifty-some magnets collected over years of awayness, displaying glossy names and sights of US states and Canadian provinces. The top goal on his bucket list was owning a magnet from every state, purchased on a trip. Only South Dakota and Alaska are missing. He and I had intended to check off South Dakota together, perhaps after the Cuba trip we also discussed. The best I can do is remove the faded magnets, round, square, and oval, and make them my prized possessions. It hurts beyond any unbearable pain to have your dad reduced to an incomplete collection of weathered US state magnets. Yet I don't have time to feel the pain.

Then I see it. On the kitchenette table, next to an ashtray and matches, I see the friggin' tube, the reason I have returned. It's a turquoise aluminum canister holding perfumed wood incense sticks, and still occupying the same spot as last Memorial Day. Its scent may say "Ocean Spray," but betrayal is what I smell. Wicked incense. Intended to calm and uplift—and not something a hardworking sixty-year-old male from Frederikshavn would ever have in mind to own. Though Mother Karin comes to Atlanta once a year, fragrances and perfumes of any sort bother her breathing.

I open the canister. Only a few sticks remain. I remove one, inhale its fake fragrance, and feel anything but calmed. For a whole year, I've been trying to deny the tube that is not our family way. I've tried to not be a truth-seeker. I've tried to favor blindness. I've tried to ignore that Magnum sometimes has a guest in the apartment, someone who uses incense sticks in the kitchen's common area, and all conclusions end up at the same bottom line: That someone is a female. The same female who uses the opened pack of menstrual pads inside a bathroom cabinet.

Favoring blindness has absolutely not worked for me. My skin is literally incensed; up and down my arms are pus-filled sores that have developed at the injection sites of my anti-anemia medication, each one appearing after our Peachtree visit last year. My skin displays the price of silencing the nagging question within, of not wanting to know what I already do know.

Except now I do. I want to know all of it.

Mother Karin likes to put a cover on things, as if life is a pot you must lid. She could have spared me a terribly burnt stew the Christmas following my first visit to New York City and Spanish Harlem when I announced that an American was joining us for the holidays. She and I were laying the long table in the dining room at Halfdansvej 9, squaring Royal Copenhagen plates evenly on the starched tablecloth. Mother Karin responded, "I hope he isn't a drug dealer."

She didn't even look up as she said this; perhaps she didn't want to witness the look of bewilderment I couldn't possibly hide. The first time Calvin was mentioned, Mother Karin intuited he was someone with a dark drug side.

Shortly after, Calvin showed up for the holidays, and he exposed Mother Karin's bathrooms to lines of white. Not that anyone caught on. Now I am here to locate something, because I don't want a lidded pot of life ever again. I want lines to be out in the open.

Times are indeed many when Mother Karin has refused to allow life to cook, boil, and turn tender with everything in open view. She has lidded anything uncomfortable—like Bodil, Uncle Frank's platinum blonde CEO wife, seducing her Magnum husband.

The weekend Mother Karin and Magnum visited Minneapolis to meet our newborn, Mother Karin and I encountered unique confidentiality, perhaps because she burst into tears when I, standing in the entryway to our apartment, removed the yellow blanket and revealed my baby girl to her mormor for the first time. This was a moment I never could have made up. "Oh she is adorable, she is beautiful, Nette," Mother Karin sniffled while I sobbed along.

The beauty of the little thing I was holding was something we at last agreed upon, and the little thing was building a way where formerly there had been none. In becoming a mother, I gained a mother. That was wonderful, real, and uncovered, a minute lasting way past the doorway where baby Dandelion bridged mother-daughter. And the following day, when a client's call had Magnum suddenly leaving for Seattle, breaking a promise to spend time with his wife on her annual US trip, Mother Karin spoke in a rare low tone that didn't match the frustration she must have been feeling.

We were both on the couch, I nursing a baby, and she nursing an intractable cough.

Magnum was always leaving and never wanted to spend time with her, she whispered between hacking. He was making her feel so lonely. And something was going on between him and Frank's wife, Bodil. Frank never came by any longer, and the abrupt chill between him and Magnum was dreadful; they'd always been great friends, amused by each other's wit.

Mother Karin was right. She and I, mother and daughter, were two people who didn't need hard evidence to know something was going on. If it was in the air, we sensed it. Besides, the Christmas before Dandelion was conceived, Bodil's red lips and red-lacquered hands had seemed to repeatedly find their way onto Magnum with coy kisses and fleeting touches at various gatherings. Having Bodil show up and find a spot next to Magnum wherever he went that holiday, hands all over him, had been an altogether new form of Christmas spirit. But in our family, no one heeded big blemishes, even new ones, and Magnum hadn't resisted the red advances of his sister-in-law.

That day when he left for Seattle, I told Mother Karin that I had observed him pressing a note into Bodil's manicured hand as she and Uncle Frank were leaving the Halfdansvej house one starlit night.

Silence. And then Mother Karin whispered she didn't know what to do.

I did: butt heads with the big blemish, better late than never, and ask Magnum. Ask him what was going on. It was about time.

I believed Mother Karin when she said that was what she was going to do—ask Magnum, for real. But somewhere she found another lid, and Bodil and Magnum's affair stayed unnamed, stewing, under cover. Because Mother Karin doesn't ever want to know.

I do.

I am in the living room by the small desk in the corner, next to a bookcase. I swallow something without a name while my hands caress the books that used to be Magnum's. It could be here. Magnum's preferred spot wasn't by the West Coast ocean. It was by a desk—books, pens, phone at the ready. A perfect spot for burying a secret.

I pull out a John Grisham novel and reach behind. Indeed, my fingers meet something hard; it turns out to be a Czech-Danish dictionary, the one Magnum had sixteen-year-old Nette bike to town to get, and also a weathered little black notebook. *I'll deal with you later*, I think at the unforgivable dictionary before dumping it in my pile and opening the black notebook. Its pages are yellowed, some frayed, and filled with quotes in a cursive pencraft that can't be taught or bought but is given—the same firm, elegant, voluptuous strokes of art that have beautified postcards crossing the globe for decades, uplifting people.

Its first entry is dated December 2, 1975—the day Magnum turned thirty-two, just about my current age.

Love is many things
A smile that springs from quiet thought
A silent voice the heart can understand
The warmth and comfort of another hand
A treasured secret told
A moment caught

Men as well as women are much more often led by their hearts than by their understanding.

In the Peachtree apartment, I suddenly beam.

"Is everything all right?" Charles speaks from the chair while lowering the paper an inch. He, too, notices how a lucky strike can cheer you, even amid calamity.

There is no Heaven like mutual Love.

God's rarest blessing is after all a good woman.

Yes, Charles. Everything's more than all right, because in this little black notebook Magnum penned beliefs, ideas. Muses touched him, and even if they weren't his original ideas, they spoke faith. Something I didn't think he harbored. Now it turns out my father was a romantic, a dreamer, someone who quoted great poets like Byron and Shakespeare. He had so much inside, even if all he let out was a trail of postcards.

Magnum was always writing. Give him a pen, typewriter, or keyboard, and he'd sit down at a desk with a coffee or gin and tonic and an ashtray and find a reason for words to flow; always small stuff, like detailed work reports, someone's CV, birthday cards, cards of any kind, and, clearly, postcards. But I always knew—and this little black notebook is the missing link—Magnum was a writer within. That was his truth. Yet life and Nanghsi would have him be a machinist, his hands to be used for labored breadwinning.

I have never felt closer to him than in this moment when I read the beginning pages in his hidden notebook, a storybook of sorts that unveils his soul to me. He wasn't faithless after all.

Then everything shifts. Damn! I turn more pages, and the sudden glow in the apartment is short-lived. Entries change; or rather, their tone changes. The scribe has turned cynical.

Maids only want husbands and when they get them they want everything.

Misogynist, even.

A wife is a woman who sticks with her husband through all the trouble he wouldn't have if he hadn't married her.

What happened? Somewhere Magnum's handsome writing stops begging the mystery of love. A hardened voice, misogynist or misogamist, loather of women or marriage, or both, moves into its place. I don't know this man. I slam the black notebook shut. Something else to deal with later.

His office. I smell it. This isn't a soulless room with things in precise rows but a space that oozes warmth and Magnum. Bookshelves hold manuals and artwork, and his trinkets from travels are scattered in corners, even lines lost. By the window overlooking the pool stands a huge mahogany desk. This is the desk of a doer, someone who needs a space to work on—lay out reports, bids—with laptop, Rolodex, cell, and camera within easy access at all times. *It's here.*

The drawers are deep, much deeper than their kin at Halfdansvej 9. My childhood dug surprising things out from drawers, items that told me things I otherwise wouldn't have known. Like the dog tag of Peter, Magnum's very best friend, who died in a motorcycle accident when they were twenty-two. Magnum held on to that dog tag forever after.

Hands tremble as I pull out the top drawer. Atop sits a fresh blue envelope loaded with family photos Magnum hasn't yet fitted into his series of albums. A mauve envelope, anything but brand-new, calls me next. I open it and feel a universal punch when I see a photo of a dark-haired, tanned woman lounging poolside. Hands won't listen and they fumble awhile before more photos follow of the same tanned, eye-splitting body of a woman in bikinis, shorts, and short skirts, each shot revealing legs to die for and curves other women pay for. White sand, boats, an "Air Jamaica" airport sign. Backgrounds sure vary, but the same woman stays the highlight. While she ages, her anatomy doesn't. The mauve reveals big, round breasts and loins covered by a small blue string. A topless shot of my father's mistress.

The explosion of reactions wanting to tumble out cannot happen, or my mission will fail, and truth will not be discovered. Anything but truth is too expensive right now. So I press on.

It takes two to make a marriage a success, and only one a failure.

I cannot fail to notice that her smile is even, white, and winning, and that she resembles a dark version of Karin in her younger days. Except the darker version is wrapping her legs and body into poses intended to lure and seduce, miles removed from Mother Karin's disposition, as far north is from way east.

I laugh. I must laugh. Magnum kept photos of a dark-haired woman who could be Mother Karin's double, if it weren't for her oomph and darkness. Life is sad and yet so heartbreakingly funny.

Then my reason for coming—the picture that answers, *Why the friggin' tube?* Her hair remains short and thick, her body language still sizzles. Even so, time shows up in lines on the hand wrapping around a coffee mug in the kitchen. The woman has been in this place, and she filled it with her ocean spray fragrance recently. That is an intrusion that ruins the feel-good warmth of Magnum's second home.

As if to confirm, the next two photos show Magnum in the apartment, dressed up for an evening out, gin and tonic in hand. This is Magnum as I last saw him—gray-haired, pale, and beaming.

Mother Karin doesn't take pictures. *She* is the reason for his beam.

When I reach the last photos in the deep stack, something bigger and more devastating than a call from a Miami-Dade detective mere hours ago bursts into the room, a miscalculation with killing power. She's wearing a short mauve dress and black stockings, wrapping youthful movie-star legs around an odd chair next to an odd lamp in an altogether odd living room. Then a young, dressed-up couple at an odd restaurant table, camera catching them head-on, Magnum—because it *is* Magnum—wearing a wide-lapelled blue suit I have no recollection of, no trace of gray in his dark mop. Bejeebers, this wasn't a fling or a brief romance. *This was a relationship lasting decades.* And *She* is no Dane or American. The odd furniture speaks of a different era and country.

Hands tremble, tremble terribly, as the next shot drops into my hand; meanwhile, all I can think is that I don't need to guess where *She*'s from.

Snap. There *She* is again, on an odd couch with two children, one little and one bigger, next to her. Life changes in a snap when you look at a little girl and realize you have a sister in a foreign country, birthed by a woman your dad has loved for twenty-some years. Loved in secret and under cover. The little girl, lighter than her sister on the couch, shares the distinct, wide brow and deep-set eyes belonging to Sister Sallie and several cousins, a unique Nilsson family trait that cannot be denied or covered up. Behind her is a pillow with the letters *O N* embroidered into it.

I have no doubt that I am looking at my father's child. Another Nilsson. Death is so revealing.

I collect the photos and place them in the mauve envelope next to me. This evidence isn't leaving my sight; it's for my eyes only. The scathe of being a truth-seeker is not something that can be imagined. Because I cannot share this. I have to keep it all inside, on my own. It would destroy my family. Lids, big blemishes—suddenly, I get them. My hands are trembling, terribly.

To make it past the stack of photos in the mauve envelope that holds my father's other life, grief leaves. It vanishes out the window into the humid Peachtree air. I don't know that I ever again will meet the grief of losing Magnum. Nor if I want to.

My hands stop trembling. I feel so empty. Then I hear Viggo's voice sweeping in from the past—Viggo, who had dark curls, blue eyes, and mischief and precociousness written all over him. We were playmates, classmates, and walk-to-school buddies. He always knew things I didn't know, which enticed me to spend many an afternoon at his home farther down Friggsvej, past Red Tomato's house. In third grade, Viggo gave me the scoop on fathers who traveled and raised a question that has been with me until now, a question that had me fly to Atlanta when really my body was too weak to go anywhere: He asked if I knew that fathers who travel have ladies wherever they go, and he asked how many my father had. He wasn't sure about the figure for his own father, who drove cargo trucks past the border. But he bet my father had a lot.

Now I have to retract the number I gave Viggo because Magnum didn't just have Mother Karin after all. The answer to the suspicion raised by a nine-year-old boy who knew much about life is way worse than the small sins—a handful of flings, a few one-night stands—that have always been my worst-case scenario.

In open view, in the second drawer, lies additional confirmation. He didn't even do us the courtesy of hiding it. On several pieces of paper, in an address book, and on a calendar, a name is written in firm, voluptuous cursive strokes. Now I know who *She* is. *She* is Magda, and it isn't only the angles of her face but also her address that confirms her Eastern European origin.

The odd connection, the strangeness sensed in a long childhood about everything Czechoslovakian, is finally established. Extended trips, calls received, a dictionary purchased, Czech crystal glasses, head-banging when Magnum wasn't at his hotel or on his way home from the Communist country few got to visit, and the three weeks when Mother Karin was hospitalized and Magnum remained working in Czechoslovakia—all were little clues, perhaps only detectable to the strong intuition of a child, a hint of Czechoslovakia always involved.

Magda lives in Olomouc, a small town in the new Czech Republic. And I am sure now that Magnum wanted us to know. *Who did you think would find your crime?* His last piece of non-bravery was letting his second daughter turn up the name, address, and photos of his other life and family. I thought I knew. But I knew nothing. Because the answer in my hand is much, much worse than anything that ever could have been conceived, even by Viggo.

Praise the art of repression, the gift bestowed by my parents. It matters not that the other life looks so goddamn happy. I move on, chill in my chest, driven by suspicion and lost loyalty.

A pile of cards and letters not in Magnum's writing beseeches me next. Despite the delay, Viggo is right, for Trinidad and Tobago, a small archipelagic state in the southern Caribbean that Magnum traveled to on business many times over the years, writes, "Happy birthday. I miss you. When are you coming again? Please call me. I love you so."

Ireland: "Hey, Sexy Sixty-year-old, cannot wait to hold you tight again."

Germany . . .

Charles moves about in the armchair, lifting the paper up and down, and my watch warns that time is too short for reading love notes from the ladies. I dump the cards in my growing pile, recalling the photos Magnum brought home from Trinidad showing people with dark skin and kinky hair, versions of Diana Ross. *Was she in any of them?* A twinge of sorriness for her hits me. She's somewhere, waiting for Magnum, who may or may not show up—another pained and powerless lady. Trinidad and Tobago, Czechoslovakia, Denmark . . . around the world, women are the same, stupidly the same.

A Western Union slip showing money wired to the Czech Republic and a sealed condom come next. More evidence. More grief that never can be claimed. How do you justify a paper route robbing childhood's last blossom when support is going way East? Just when I think there's no more to be lost, nothing else to be gone, I find the little piece of paper rounding up my inheritance. Atop stacks of gratuitous notepads from hotel chains, I see a worn sheet of paper with Magnum's curvaceous handwriting penned onto it. A brown heading says, "Ramada," and below is a matrix, a table neatly drawn in pencil with clear, even lines. Each cell is filled in; the sheet brims with names. Female names. Next to each name is a location abbreviation and a number. Sonya DK 1, Bjørk N 3, Paula UK 300, Marsha US 2, Magda CZ 1000.

It takes a little time to sink in, but this is . . . a scorecard.

A scorecard. My father kept a scorecard, not of the local baseball team in Atlanta or his favorite soccer club since childhood but of the women he'd screwed. I take a closer look. Magda CZ has the highest score, by far. There are several things here that would repulse me, were I able to feel. Some entries have no name: *Tr To 1*—a nameless screw in Trinidad and Tobago? Was she so unimportant he didn't bother to get her name? *Ger 1*—same thing, another nameless fuck in Germany. Several more unnamed tallies. *Bodil DK*, no score, is a newer entry, indicated by its lower position on the page. Must be an entry for my aunt, logged after that Christmas. Couldn't he make up his mind about her? *Cz, Cz, Cz*—numerous names with Czech entries. Magda wasn't enough. Had to try other sisters in the land, huh? *Flight to DK 1.* No wonder he often told Karin not to bother getting him at the airport, pretending to spare her the effort when in actuality, he knew he might be busy finishing a screw with a happenstance flight encounter. Where? In the bathroom? In empty seats? In a corner of the Copenhagen airport only he knew of?

And then the entry that makes me fatherless: *Fatso DK 1.* As my eyes fall on this recorded fuck, I decide I no longer have a father. The man who had insisted on, vehemently insisted on, and enforced no name-calling in our household was referring to a woman, someone he'd put his dick into, as Fatso. Mother Karin is right. He did have an abhorrence of fat people. Screw her, use her, and then call her Fatso.

You are not *my father. In the name of women—the women you have screwed, the women you wanted to screw, the women you were going to screw, dots of women around the world in places you visited—I denounce you as my father.*

This moment, I say STOP—for all of us, for those who can't.

How many times can you lose a father? Apparently, one last time, the ultimate, irretractable last time. The loss of all. Except it feels like no loss.

I breeze through the rest of the office. I've found what needs to be found. The dead man had primed the job for me by placing all evidence in the spot where people who knew him would look: his desk drawers.

In the living room, I tell Charles that I am done.

"That was quick. We'll have plenty of time to get back to the airport." In a gentle voice, he adds, "You'd make your dad proud. He'd be so proud you're doing this. You have such strength!"

All at once, I remember Mother Karin's only request. In the hallway, near the entry, is a closet; I walk across to peek into its dimness. His set, a black stand bag loaded with golf clubs, rests in a corner. But there is no pink set purchased by the dead man for his wife.

"Would you mind checking the Jeep for a pink golf set?" I ask. "It's supposed to be here somewhere."

Charles gets up and heads outside. They were going to start golfing because that's what you do in Frederikshavn when you're past sixty, middle-class, and retired. Mother Karin has long been itching to wheel a unique set of pink American golf clubs around the tees before fellow hometowners.

That won't be happening.

"I'm sorry, but it's not there," Charles says, huffing, as he returns from the hot parking lot. "The car's empty."

I nod. I know where the pink clubs are. In the other life.

I look in the closet again. A heavy professional toolbox meets my glance. That was his. I recognize it and have known its shape since I was a toddler. Specialty tools for a working man, gadgets I don't know the name of. The contents of the box are worth a lot of money. Instead of her pink golf set, Mother Karin will get Magnum's toolbox.

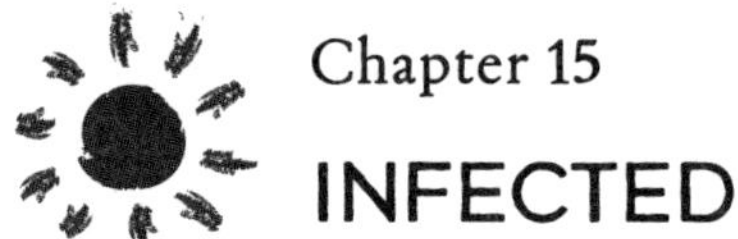

Chapter 15
INFECTED

June has almost come and gone. On the last day of the month, I am on a lawn chair in a corner of Mother Karin's manicured green; the sun above is my only companion. The funeral is tomorrow. The kitchen is filled with bereavement—people coming and going, tears, bouquets in all sizes, incomprehension, and a blanket of thick grief that wraps around all who knew Mag. Mother Karin is the new centerpiece.

There is so much to accept and forgive. I want to throw up—gag life out on the perfect grass, retch away all that I must accept. And forgive. My body can stand no more burdens. For the sake of my health, I have to find forgiveness for the dead man and accept the false show in the kitchen of people who don't know. They worship the jolly man who sent postcards, unaware that hiding in his drawers was a screwing scorecard and a stack of blank cards bought in shops around the globe. If they look closer, they will notice that their cards weren't always sent from Abu Dhabi or San Diego but were often postmarked in Atlanta. Postcards were a convenient cover when Magnum didn't want to be available for his family because he'd rather spend time with his mistress, or whatever you call someone your dad shared a life, a home, and children with for nearly thirty years. *Wife Two?* I don't have a name for what the man has done.

I roll up my pants to look at my legs. This morning, I awoke with an odd sensation in several spots on my shins, and as the day progressed, the stinging spots have broken open, oozing pus. They look far from good. The red lesions appear to be deepening each time I check. They are telling me something: I am infected with a lie, or however you label the perfidiousness of the man, the master liar, Mag.

Mag spoke Czech. Not just a few broken words or failed sayings; he mastered a fluency that enabled him to negotiate a Skoda car deal for family two and also made it possible for him to take Magda's oldest daughter to the hospital, where he told doctors what happened when a key set hit her forehead and she needed stitches. Learning Czech is almost as hard as learning Chinese for a Germanic-speaking person. I know so because Cal—who is so gifted that he can learn a language nearly overnight—failed. Before the trip we took to Prague during our year in Copenhagen, he gave learning Czech an intense whirl. We both expected he'd be shooting the bull with locals in their native tongue in no time, but it was too hard, even for him.

I get now that when I overheard Magnum in the kitchen answering calls coming from under the Iron Curtain, it wasn't broken syllables he was uttering but Czech for real. He spoke with the kind of language intelligibility that demands extraordinary skill, effort, and will to learn.

Magda doesn't speak English, save a few words. She does know a bit of Italian. This I know because I've sort of talked to her, and she let me know that Mag had to learn Czech or they wouldn't have a way to communicate. Speaking Czech was perhaps Mag's biggest joke. He fooled us all.

The afternoon I left Charles in the Atlanta airport and arrived home in Seaside past midnight, I got out of the cab and went into my house, lugging a heavy suitcase full of Magnum's belongings. Despite the strange vacancy in my chest, the trip was all worth it. *No more lies*. And, *She must have loved him*. I couldn't let Magda linger in the unknown, not grasping why Mag didn't answer or come or wire money again. I couldn't let him be gone for no reason. I couldn't let her suffer. *She needs to know*. My compassion toward the dark-haired woman was a mystery even to myself.

That same night, I dialed her number. We stumbled through the introduction, but eventually, my Latin and her Italian met up, and a few shared English words helped us through a brief conversation. I told her Nils was gone for good. Between suppressed sobs, she let me know she'd spoken to him a few days earlier and that she already had a ticket for her next visit to Atlanta. She knew enough words to let me know Nils spoke Czech. She wanted me to write. Her daughter knew *poco* English. We were two foreign voices sharing an understanding that cannot be categorized.

When we hung up, I didn't feel much of anything, except the comfort of having done the right thing by calling. Sometime in the future, I will learn that Magda didn't share my absence of emotions and had, in fact, blacked out on the living room floor when our call ended. In a future dialogue, she will tell me Nils had a big heart because he loved two families.

Are you fucking kiddin' me?

I know why he died. Two women both pulling at him to retire—a double life with an impossible ending. The ending he couldn't pull off; the rest, yeah, but he couldn't give them both the finale they demanded in the last segment of life, not without the cover of his job. Maybe he didn't want to, either. His heart gave in or gave up, torn into two sorry stories that never would make a happy whole. In the end, good and happy were impossible with two families at once. That took him thirty years to figure out.

From the lawn chair, nothing matters. I am utterly exhausted from seeking, finding, and handling truth. The lesions are urgent signals, the manifestations of a war within—a war where I am a surprising opponent who has added the worst betrayal of all. That is who I am in this exhausted lawn moment. My own enemy.

I couldn't do it to Mother Karin and my siblings. I could neither show nor tell the inheritance Mag left us in Atlanta, the betrayal in his drawer. It is enough that one of us is infected with a lie. Honesty would only destroy. The irony is that I have told Wife Two but not Wife One. Mother Karin gets spared, and so does Magda, each in their own way. I am the only one who isn't reprieved.

A few days ago, I finally showed Mother Karin the things I brought from the Peachtree apartment. She was only interested in the little brown address book Magnum meticulously kept for years.

I didn't flinch when Mother Karin accepted her husband's book of contacts, and anxious words fell out of her: "I don't want to know . . . are there any names in it?"

Two pages lined with Czech names and addresses were missing—removed and left in my desk in Seaside. So I didn't lie when I answered, "No, there are no names."

"Thank God. I was so afraid." She reached for the address book that once would have told her everything and dumped it into a drawer. Its life was over. Then a puzzled look overcame her, as if something was missing or a missing question was dared. "It's odd, don't you think, about the golf set? Where could he have put it? He bought it for me. He told me so."

"Yes, it's odd," I acknowledged aloud. *It's no friggin' mystery. Magda has a set of nice pink golf clubs back home in Olomouc. And you know! You fucking know.*

Mother Karin's lips quivered. "Did . . . did you find anything else in the apartment? Anything I wouldn't want to know about?"

The loyal child answered with lips of steel, "No, I didn't."

It was in that instant that I turned enemy to myself. I missed my opportunity to once and for all right the ways of our family, to blow lids, blemishes, and cover stories away with truth. Instead, to shield others from what they didn't want to know—even if they already did—I covered up, and I harmed myself by going against the principle of *No more lies*.

That contradiction kills my legs. My own betrayal is too much to bear. On the lawn chair, separated from the ongoing kitchen spectacle, I am still learning the prize of needing more answers, of urging the universal nudge to keep on hurling force. I crave as much truth as possible. I crave it all—so that I may forgive in an unknown future.

Mere hours ago, I dug into the laptop that accompanied Mag everywhere. Mother Karin had asked me to look for a Canadian bank account. He'd once mentioned opening one. Just as he had once emailed me from a Yahoo! account, not from his shared marital email or work account. A Yahoo! account was then akin to Mag using ChatGPT, not something a hardworking man from the north adopts. This email was a rare slip, and my keen eye caught the small infraction. A two-line message a couple of years ago from a Yahoo! account—that was my reason for getting on Mag's laptop and looking for more answers.

The Canadian savings account remains anonymous for now, although Magda will later confirm, via a friend translating, that she and Mag were house-hunting in Vancouver. He was stashing away for retirement—perhaps in a Canuck account, but with a Czech cosigner.

That doesn't matter to me on this day before the funeral, but the Yahoo! account does.

A few hours ago, without thinking, I typed a password into the Yahoo! home page and received a flashing error message. I sank back into the chair. I had to get this!

Two tries were left. Then I knew what to do. I connected upward, or wherever the direction to the divine is, and I besought password help. In that one moment, I was one with the direction, and it returned. A Yahoo! account soon opened on the small screen.

The email inbox was empty, but the dead man had a fully stocked dating profile, seeking any female within a fifty-mile radius of Atlanta. No discrimination on his part, regardless of ethnicity, body type, religion, or marital status—anything went. The only restriction was age; he preferred women who were just a hair older than his oldest daughter but slightly younger than his wife, Karin. *How could he?* One wife, two wives, the list of women scored on his travels weren't enough? He had to womanize, screw around, whore when he was in Atlanta, his second home? His betrayal—his lack of loyalty to women, to *any* woman—seemed boundless and wicked. Yet, before I had a chance to notice the nausea striking me, irony budded into the office and had me shake my head in a mix of bewildered laughs and almost-tears. The password! The password used to enter his whoring account was none other than the name of his original wife: Karin.

If it's possible to be stranded in an upstairs office, what used to be your home, as if you're the clichéd "only survivor" of a shipwreck on a deserted island, I just managed to do that.

Who was this man?

My life until now has been a sham.

Who am I?

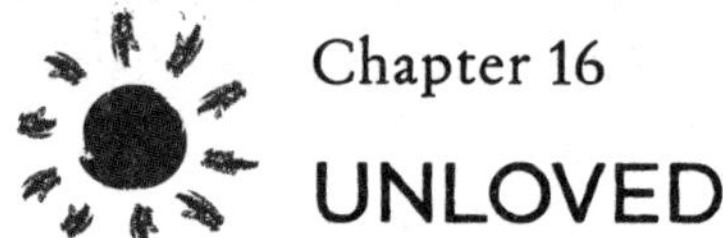

Chapter 16

UNLOVED

The scorecard haunts me.

I've fled my biological family. They're not to be trusted. Back in Seaside, Denmark is a bad memory I absconded from after a family trip to Luxembourg in a van holding Mother Karin, Sister Sallie, Leif, three young kids, and myself, but no Mag to hold everyone together. Mere days after his funeral, the rented van clocked hundreds of kilometers on European motorways to get us to and from a baptism for baby Simon Nils. The trip was a nightmare lasting a week. For no apparent reason other than years of unspoken sentiments not of a happy and good nature, tension followed the van to and from Penis and Poline's home. For once, Mother Karin and I were in the same camp—opposing Sister Sallie and Leif—while the kids suffered in the middle, a family traveling together but not talking.

Sometimes, truth isn't found but released. When the van returned everyone to Halfdansvej, unspoken tension hidden under a long cover story finally gave way to exploding vitriol inside the hallway of Mother Karin's home. Ignited by the bag of Haribo sweets Aunt Sallie handed Dandelion—another bag I didn't want her to have—in a split second, my sister and I were at each other's throat, shoving, screaming, and hurling insults and sincerity while struggling to gain power over the van keys. This was a tussle about much more than who got to drive off. Spit, tears, and body spatter of all sorts whirled while Mother Karin and the kids' shocked faces watched a duke-out unlike any ever seen in an upstanding family in the north.

Such enmity doesn't happen in an instant. This was a fight that should have been years ago; its deferment only made it more vicious. But these weren't normal times. In normal times, I would have struck down my sister in one fast, decisive move and grabbed the keys out of her hand, just as the father I have disowned would have stalled the fight, stopped two sisters from swinging hurt and hate at each other. He would have stopped Sister Sallie from yelling all the reasons I was an unfit mother, abusing my child with my ways, my angry eyes, my illness that wasn't getting any better, and my refusal to do something about it. Everything was diminished, not normal, and my body—gone to lesions—couldn't act normal. I couldn't stop Sister Sallie from yelling she was going to call Social Services on me. I couldn't stop knowing she would make good on her malice because that was her way. But I could stop the call that would have me lose my daughter.

It just can't happen. I released myself from the fight and made my weak legs scramble up the stairs. Inside my former bedroom, I locked the door. Sallie tailed my unforeseen move and was banging on the door in seconds. Below in the hallway, Mother Karin was finally shouting, "Stop it! Stop it!"—years overdue and yet another ineffectual motion, like head-banging, that got no one anywhere.

Fortified behind a secure door, I turned Sallie's own weapon on her and dialed the police to report that my sister wouldn't let me leave.

Shaking from rage, I didn't know what to think, so I simply followed orders and handed the cell phone to Sallie through a cracked-open door. The authoritative voice easily swayed her to surrender the car keys and fight.

Now I am back in New York, less a father, a sister, a home, and heaven knows what else.

I do have my daughter. She still sleeps next to me in the lime-green sheets, and that's precious. But the fight that made me call the cops on my sister this summer is a truth I don't want to know. What's still unknown to me—I have so much to learn in the days ahead—is that dirt must come out in order to heal the inside. The fight between Sallie and me may seem, feel, and look like an irreparable setback, yet our physical altercation is really a step forward. Perhaps if we'd hurled and released sooner or oftener, we wouldn't be two sisters with holes in our guts, resorting to the authorities to handle one another.

The summer in Denmark has left my body a festering monster, my heart broken and ashamed, and now a question mark envelops me: *Who are we?*

The three weeks I spent in a Danish hospital after I fled in the van was good for something. The Danish docs—each one more handsome than the last in the big hospital in the north—said they'd rarely seen a worse case of Crohn's, but they could fix me. Surgery was the way to go. Just like Sister Sallie, equipped with an ostomy bag and quality of life, I was fixable. The fresh linens of a hospital in the north, docs you call by their first name, and the presence those docs bring to your room don't come any finer. I told them I would think about it. What I really was thinking about was Sallie. She had been speaking a truth the day when Social Services and the police entered our lives. My daughter was suffering unintended abuse by way of illness.

My sister was right. *Dandelion deserves so much better.*

That's why I am back in New York. I've gone looking for the two people who will help fix me—because no knife is going to cure me. It can't. For a time, maybe, but then the festering will return, and another knife will be needed. I wish this weren't so. I wish the pleading docs were right: stay, receive our care, and get well. How easy that would be, resting in the fresh white linens. But the illness inside me isn't simply a piece of colon that can be surgically removed and forgotten about. Healing isn't always a straight line following bed rest; sometimes, it follows a twisted trajectory, especially when seeking truth is involved.

Yet something has to give. Now. My girl needs much more than a joyless, hushed parenting figure for whom everything is obviously a chore, my illness not a guest but a presence that clings like foul halitosis, something she can't ignore for it escapes every time her mama breathes, sullying whatever it touches—sullying her entire childhood.

Enough is enough, and I need to find the missing piece, the reason why my physical condition isn't improving. I am haunted by not knowing anything but the physical leftovers from someone who scored his infidelity sex with women—and left the scorecard for his second child to discover. Knowing the truth isn't just knowing evidence surrendered in a drawer. Not knowing the motive for the evidence, this truth is nearly worthless. To truly know the truth, I need to find the whys for the scorecard: the double life and the story that was our family.

That's why I will meet my spiritual parents this fall morning after the yellow school bus has picked up Dandelion. They see straight through me, into me. They see why my body remains out of control. They know the answers to the distress that made Mag pen *Fatso* on a hotel pad with *1* written next to it, surrounded by other scores—full disclosure in death, no mercy. They will tell me straight-up—no cuddling, tough details—what is really going on in me, in my family, behind the scenes, and will tell me which non-physical matters are causing this physical havoc. Judgment is a word they don't know when you sit with them. They are firm love-holders who only have given me a reason to trust. And I do, with Foster and Kristos, *I do*. Foster, you already know. Kristos was added a while ago. He's built like a bull, with classical Greek features and penetrating Aegean blue eyes, as if he is a statue that belongs in the National Archaeological Museum of Athens—yet he was raised in Germany and is now Foster's life partner. He cannot be labeled, categorized, or explained. Sometimes, gifts are so unique that they bear no name. Such is the case with Kristos, though Foster introduced his partner as a "medical intuitive" when I first met him a few seasons ago. It's as if Kristos has an open file on your body, your psyche, your past, your family, and everything you have ever encountered, the things you know and don't know, and he directs you to particulars in the file that you need to hear in order to move on, to heal. He's also someone who read twenty versions of the Bible at once, including the Aramaic, to see for himself how the life of the Bible has evolved into a story far removed from its origin. Though Kristos is a facilitator for the realm beyond Earth, his self-education in matters of the physical world is mastery itself. He knows what he is talking about, always. He's my kind of guy.

When I am out of options, and my body yells at me to get a grip, to get cured, and I have no one to lean on but a knife I don't trust, these are the two men I seek. Foster and Kristos are the medicine surgeons who will help me cut out, remove, and heal the festering inside. They speak in a way I know, even when I don't, and I have always left strengthened, straightened, and a better version of myself after I have sat with them.

TODAY, WE'RE MEETING on the East End in a huge mansion belonging to another client. In the dark living room where my spiritual parents await me, a soft breeze blows through an open window, seducing a curtain into billowing playfully against the intruding waft. It feels good, even if my body doesn't.

Foster is sitting cross-legged on a mat. Soon, I'm next to him with Kristos, who sits erect like a chiseled statue in a luxury leather armchair before us—a veritable chic advertisement were he not wearing budget flip-flops. He hasn't fully shaken off the poverty of an immigrant childhood in Nuremberg.

"What do you want to work on?" Foster asks. His shamanic healing tools lie next to him, placed with care and reverence in exact rows. I welcome their nearness and the work ahead of them. I welcome this moment.

"It's been an awful summer . . . my . . . dad died . . . turned out he led a secret life. I have questions about that."

A deep exhale of prana leaves Kristos. He shifts into the gift of his gaze and speaks: "See, Nette, how revealing death can be? All the hidden stuff comes up. It's a tradition in your family not to reveal." Pause. "Your dad made a choice because he couldn't take his life anymore—the hypocrisy, the lies. His heart gave up. He chose to die rather than reveal. The problem now"—Kristos is still a newcomer to America, and he halts to find the right expression—"is who is left behind has to deal with the secrets and—"

"No one knows but me!" I interrupt.

"Everyone knows to some degree," he says mildly.

He's right. Of course, they know. During our last family dinner at Halfdansvej 9, Mag pondered aloud how he was going to swing another trip back home for Mother Karin's upcoming birthday. If the tax man found out, he'd lose the 180-day benefit. As she dumped a well-done pork chop on his plate, Mother Karin provided the answer: "Just tell them you're going to see your mistress. That should get you off scot-free." When the table was cleared for dessert, sound returned to the kitchen, and Mag stopped shaking his head.

"You see, they do." Kristos captures my attention again. "There's a silent acceptance, even if your mother pretends not to know. That's your mother's choice. Because, as hard as it is accepting a mistress, the alternative would be harder. Your dad was the hero in her world, mistress or no mistress." The intruding waft reaches the floor, cooling the delivery of his gaze.

Of course! Unbeknownst to herself, Mother Karin taught me hero worship. Her one unequivocal deed was adoring the man she married, even if she couldn't help the misery she and he added to their marriage. She had good reason to wait thirty-some years to spend time with her husband, her hero.

"I miss him so!" For months, since I lost a father I didn't know, I have not felt anything but numbness when the jolly man has come to mind. Grief seemed forever gone—until now. That's the thing with Foster and Kristos: They put you in direct contact with a place where things you can't sense dwell. Your innermost sanctuary. Where heroes rest.

"Yes," Kristos says, "but you see, he says, 'You missed me already when I was there.'"

So true. I've always missed him, and I still do.

"Cry, honey, do cry," Kristos encourages me. "You'll get over it. Your dad says, 'I just gave up. There was no value in continuing. All I did was work, function, and create a double life.'"

"But he spread so much joy to other people! That's invaluable!" I say through sniffles that won't stop.

"He did, absolutely. But he says, 'Just because I brought joy doesn't mean I was joyful.'"

No! How could that be?

Yet I know it is true. My big, brawny father wasn't jolly. The jolly man—another deception. Maybe they weren't false signals—those fleeting sad expressions caught on Mag in moments when he thought he was alone: behind the newspaper or with his back turned, making a dark pot of coffee.

Why didn't he share his hurt? Why didn't he let us help him? Why did he always pretend?

I needn't ask. Kristos is ahead of my question. "It wasn't that he was a fake. He didn't want to be a burden, emotionally. He couldn't really reveal to someone what was going on inside of him, that he had a deep problem. He had never learned the skills to admit to a problem. That is why the working mode was so important for him."

A note from the future: The expectation of heroes needs to change. Let showing your vulnerability and your aches with your family be a true hallmark of a hero. Let us honor the men who show and share their hurt in accountable ways. No drawers necessary. We will all benefit. For man's wounds and man's powers spring from the same place. How can a hero know his power if he doesn't know his wound?

On the mat before Kristos and Foster, six-year-old Nils jumps to mind. I picture a gentle boy easily brought to tears, forced to deliver loads of newspapers to a large neighborhood each morning when others were still sleeping. Farmor Nanghsi wasn't the merciful kind. Nils's earnings had to be handed over every payday. Farmor claimed she needed his help to get rye bread and pork fat on the dinner table. In return, Nils became a breadwinner at the mere age of six, turning away from tears and into someone who never after had a sick day, someone whose ability to provide superseded everything else in him. So much loss for a simple dinner. A childhood's full blossom clipped and handed over. Yet he found a way to bring home more than earnings, to be a joy-maker. With a robbed childhood and lost dreams in the face of so much potential and yearning, isn't that something? No doubt Dandelion would relish some of the jolly man in her mother these days.

Something remains unclear to me: "What was his problem?"

"He had to deal with a great doubt in his mind," Kristos answers. "He had a certain kind of melancholy; it was a great issue in his soul. He says he has been fighting it for the last thirty years, but no one noticed because he was so active. The women were part of the melancholy. You see, Nette, he couldn't commit. Your mother knew that. She agreed to some degree, and he continued womanizing because it was a way to get what she couldn't give him. Your mother had no space for a husband, a lover, for sharing. It was more living side by side—in a nice house, mind you. Your dad decided to get attention from other women. But it didn't work because he had this depression, this gloom, inside. The women weren't even an addiction. He was on a search, looking for something, and he didn't know what it was."

Really! What Mag wanted was someone to share his notebook with, and all he got was a head-banging wife who wanted trophies like a rare Persian rug, bought through the awayness of her husband. A longing for a true partner made him go looking all over the globe. Looking in vain.

Through the open window, a bird is doing a solo improv, as if riffing a sympathetic song to express all that now runs through me on the mat. Once more, Mag isn't who I thought he was. There are still unopened drawers in his desk.

Kristos answers my next question. "The problem is that he met a woman who fell completely in love with him." Pause. "But he couldn't commit. He tried but couldn't."

Something terrific occurs to me. *It wasn't Magda who received Mag's last call. Mother Karin did. Thank goodness, he didn't love the other woman more.*

"The other problem is that he didn't love your mother. He respected her, he married her, and he stayed with her. But there was no love. He was looking for some kind of love that never happened. The word is, 'A mistake.' He thought he would help her change. But she was impossible to receive love from, and she never changed. That basically damaged your family. It gave him the idea, 'You are not enough. Whatever you do, it is not enough.' He says clearly he couldn't be a person who said, 'Screw you, I'm leaving.' He cared too much, out of loyalty."

How dare he claim loyalty! I know she was tough to love, but there were also three young kids who needed a father while he was away somewhere with number two in Czechoslovakia or with unknown scores in unnamed places. More than anything, we needed a fatherly buffer against Mother Karin's variety of bad habits. He got to leave her, and we didn't. Talk about a real mistake. That wasn't loyalty but cowardice. Injustice finds its way back to me.

Kristos is ahead of me once more and answers before my mental outburst can catapult into the room. "He regrets it." The sentence slides into the cool waft, words and air merging into a short reprieve. "Your mother wished him away many times and said, 'Come back. Go away.' That was her pattern. And your dad says, 'A lot of women came to me and told me I was wonderful and other things I never heard before.' This is what he was looking for and what took him away from the family. What he regrets, like death only will have you regret, is that you had to pay the price."

His regrets don't help me. Some things are just too late. I am still stuck with a poison inside. I cry out, "What hurts me the most is that I found a scorecard of women he was with, with a name, a city, and a number next to it." *Explain that one.*

No pause is needed.

"For him, it was a possibility to see how much somebody liked him," Kristos says. "The number wasn't how great the sex was, but how much he felt liked."

"Okay . . . so it wasn't . . . not the number of times he was with . . . or how good—"

"No," Kristos interrupts firmly, changing everything about the inheritance in the top drawer in my dad's desk in Atlanta.

Dizziness seizes the mat and me. I don't know that I can keep up with any more alterations to my life, the cover story, who we are, and who my dad was. Now, I really don't know who he was. That's a lot to hold. I am just one person, holding it all. I am out of storage space.

"It's an emotional rating system, basically," Kristos adds wryly, his way of confirming the comedy of a life that was my dad's. "Very inventive."

"*Okaaay* . . ." I process aloud. "That's why next to Magda, the Czech sweetheart, he'd made one number and then changed it to a thousand. The others were one, two, thirty. My aunt a nothing."

There's some justice, after all. Laughing bounces into the room, coming from three people sharing life and man at his strangest, both his worst and best self. The hilarity is a welcome change.

My dad kept a love tally, not a callous score of screws accomplished. Very low marks abounded, sadly. He made love to the whole world without ever feeling loved. Though not for a lack of trying.

In the sadness and comicality of it all, my dad has me happy one last time. Despite his many betrayals, he never sold out on the first entries in his little black notebook, on the beginning and end of all.

Kristos confirms my thoughts: "Love. He was on a search for love. Love."

Foster breaks in with a question: "What about physically? Will Nette recover?" He's asking for my benefit what he already knows.

"Your spiritual body is in turmoil," Kristos says. "Your body says, 'I am out of control, I am out of order.' Of course it is. I would only expect it to be after what you experienced." He halts a moment before continuing. "Still, when a physical condition doesn't get any better, there must be a spiritual reason, a mental reason. In your case, basically your body is your tool to push you over the edge. To change. You have been a bit of a slow learner. But you will come out stronger on the other end."

"I don't need my body as a tool anymore." *That's why I am here. To make it stop, to make it be better.*

"Your body does not do what your mind understands," Kristos explains simply. "You are on your spiritual path, but your body has yet to catch up to that. That's the nature of the physical world; it has to catch up, whether we like it or not."

I have not one but two screwed-up parents and a truly screwed-up life story.

I close my eyes and sense Foster picking up his tools to begin a shaman's clearing on my body and spirit on the mat. I've gotten what I came looking for. Truth offers change. Everything has indeed changed; most of all, my perspective has moved on. The roar of truth has come with understanding. I don't hate my father any longer. That's an enormous balm, as if all the bumblebees of the world have joined to make a special collection for me, and everything is all right.

I don't know about tomorrow, because there's a lot of catching up to do, but right now, on this mat, I am all right. I am off the trail of untruthfulness.

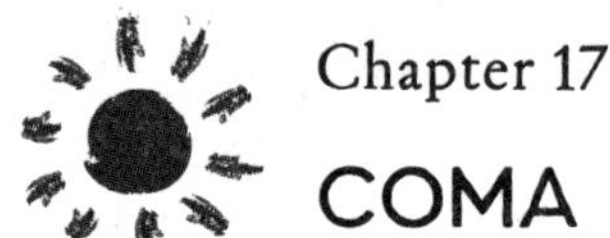

Chapter 17
COMA

In the stark silence, her caress reaches me and strokes me with its incredible tenderness. Her voice is melting, soulful, a breath of love.

You think I'd leave your side baby
You know me better than that
You think I'd leave you down

The floor is cold. My forehead rests on the crumbling bathroom tile, which I have yet to replace. I don't know where the rest of my body is. Something akin to darkness encloses me.

When you're down on your knees
I wouldn't do that

Her quiet song is soothing. It stops me from slipping away from the coldness.

I'll tell you you're right when
You want
And if only you could see into me

Dandelion is two feet away, curled up in the doorway. She cannot get any closer. An unbendable body takes up the small bathroom floor next to her. She continues her lullaby silently. Her mother has been sleeping for so long. She is worried. Scared, really.

Oh, when you're cold
I'll be there
Hold you tight to me

"*Mor*, look what I got. A chocolate bear!"

Her voice is gleeful. It reaches me through the fluffy darkness I lie within.

I must answer. Tell her how wonderful her Christmas calendar treat is. The candy surprise makes her day; that is why I bought it for her. But I can't get up. I push, but there is nothing to push. No body.

When you're on the outside
Baby and you can't get in
I will show you you're so much
Better than you know

Dandelion doesn't go downstairs again. Her mama didn't get up. The chocolate bear is gone, eaten a long time ago. She continues her whisper next to the unbending body. Her room is safe, a step away from the bathroom, and in brief breaks, she plays in there. She's still wearing her nightgown.

When you're lost, and you're alone
And you can't get back again

The darkness is gone. Bliss—pure bliss—is here in its stead. A feeling that cannot be conveyed. A luminous stream of soft, golden incandescence, that is what I am, lovingness, formidable. Grace. I see the decrepit body that is—used to be—me lying on the tile. *Why would I ever want to go back?*

I will find you, darling
and I'll bring you home

I still hear her song, her breath, her soul. She has been singing for so long. Not hours, but days. To me. Without bathroom breaks or eating or drinking. She's just six. Small and fragile. She needs . . . so much. Christmas calendars for many more years. How I yearn to leave fully, to pass through the threshold and follow the path of the golden incandescence, to lose all relation to the world of the bathroom floor and crumbling tile. An irresistible pull.

I don't want to go back. I *don't* want to go back.

And if you want to cry
I am here to dry your eyes

She is not giving up on the half-naked, rigid body that is her mama. She never thinks to leave.

Suddenly, she does not have to.

And in no time
You'll be fine
Mama

A key in the front door, and then Belle's kind voice speaks—"Anyone home?"

In no time, Jim, sirens, flashing lights, policemen, firemen, EMTs, quick footsteps up and down the stairs, frantic voices, a gurney, mask, needles, tubes, and an ambulance speeding down the Boulevard.

Oh when you're low
I'll be there
By your side baby

Before the frenzy and before Belle slips her away to the safety of the house next door, my Dandelion sings quietly for me one last time. Preciously. So I won't forget.

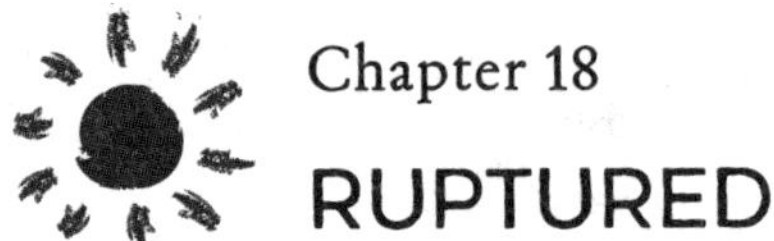

Chapter 18

RUPTURED

I am so cold. A voice shouts my name over and over, adding to the freeze. Its grating sound is low, a faint wave moving at a distance.

"Are you there? Nette, are you there?"

I don't want to hear it. But I do. Bliss is gone, and now is an irritating male voice that must belong to Jim. My eyes want to stretch into the incandescence, as if it has left a spark to clutch onto. They want to avoid the ministrations that have been going on for hours. I don't want to open my eyes to my second chance.

Another faintness: "Ms. Nilsson . . . hypothermia . . . coma . . . don't know if she . . ."

The lights are awful. An intrusion of harshness strikes from all directions, and my eyelids flicker against the blurriness. Why does my neighbor keep yelling at me? I want to shout, "Shut up," but I can't find my voice. I can't see. I can't speak. I am so cold.

Then, suddenly, a naked bulb in a ceiling emerges, as if a switch has been toggled on. As does the middle-aged face of a male who isn't Jim.

The stranger grabs my arm. "Welcome." Pause. "You had us scared, Nette."

I sigh and turn my head.

"What are *you* doing here?" With a smack's force, my vision is no longer struggling, and I see Cal on a chair. The sound coming out of me is a croak, yet the tone is irrefutable. I haven't seen my ex for months, not since I banned him from Dandelion's life. Leaving our daughter at a strange man's pool in Miami to go get more drugs, with Liam running to and from the bathroom, was my reason. If sound could kill, Cal would be keeling over this minute.

Welcome to the world.

Jim's double chortles.

Cal looks into my face with sobriety, another stranger, and speaks softly. "You are in the hospital. You are very sick." He wrings his hands and continues: "You are at St. Mary's. In the ER. You have been in a coma . . . for days."

I attempt a hiss—"Stop lying"—but the naked bulb in a drab ceiling and linens that aren't lime green do tell me I am not where I thought I was. Jim's white coat double leaves. Nothing makes sense. Not this place again. *Please.*

An older nurse with a gray pageboy cut I recall from somewhere appears. Her lips are pursed, another striking intrusion: "Don't speak. You're on a respirator. Dr. Hunter has ordered the tubes removed."

There's nothing gracious about being received by an efficient nurse with frigid hands pulling tubes out of a raw throat when you have just come back from a place of boundless light. Being assailed by a nurse who only has business on her mind is another awful entry into this world.

I am at St. Mary's. "Where's Dandelion?" I'm trying to make pieces fit but can't. I may be cold, but I don't feel like someone who's just been in a coma, someone who's very sick. It just doesn't make sense.

"She's with Belle." Cal's still wringing his hands, tanned from Florida. "You're lucky. If it weren't for those neighbors of yours . . ."

The nurse is back, interrupting with another frigid order. "They want you to have a CAT scan." She squeezes an IV bag on a pole next to me, as if speaking to it.

"No," I answer.

"*No*?" The gray-haired nurse looks at me tartly. "Why?"

"I don't need one." This piece does make sense. Doctors and hospitals are always trying to give you something you don't need; it's their training, fear, or liability, who knows? I don't need their protocol. Ever.

"You're very sick." The clipped voice continues down a trail that's not conforming to any hospital procedures, so must be stirred by a private irk. "Do you realize your luck? We didn't think you'd make it. You arrived with the body temp of a deceased person. We've been working on you for four hours—and you won't have a CAT!" The gray-haired nurse rattles off more medical details to someone whose brain has been on cold storage for days.

"It's Wednesday, December 7," Cal says when the nurse finishes. "Belle found you this morning at around 8:00 a.m. It's past noon now." He adds, "It's 2005."

I don't like what's creeping up on me. *How can it be Wednesday?* That's three days I don't know, that I haven't lived. My last vivid memory occurred on Sunday. It turned out Kristos's assessment didn't hold—or maybe it did. Maybe my body has been catching up like never before since I left him and Foster, becoming an unutterably pained, enfeebled, inflamed mess. Its dire state made me see Dr. Holmberg on Friday, five days ago. This time, I was truly asking for help.

"Please help me—remove the sickness," I begged Doc H, a tall chief surgeon at a neighboring hospital. During office visits, he usually entertains me with tales from the OR and his distant family in Copenhagen. By the time I went to him last week, he'd prescribed me the full treatment arsenal available, including chemo drugs and opioid painkillers. And that day, his schedule was overbooked.

"I don't know," he said when I showed up with my difficultness. "I think you just need to hang out at McDonald's for a few days. Get some meat on those bones." And off he went, rushing to stardom in the OR to save a guy with a chicken bone or some other item lodged in his esophagus.

Now I am here. That's where trusting docs got me. Doc H's medical advice still rankles like a punch, or worse.

On Friday, I went home and attempted to eat as the doc ordered—not a burger but some bits of a different, more wholesome protein. The protein didn't like my body, or my body didn't like the protein, however, because a mad inferno surged in my belly, bringing me to my knees on the couch on Sunday. Dandelion was somewhere in the house, playing in solitude with the princesses and other characters. I didn't know what to do. Nothing ever worked. I could bear no more. I was out of trying. And out of will. The road to tomorrow was an impossibility.

In that reckoning, something seized me. I melted into the leather and begged for help. Not from a doctor, Kristos, or myself; I begged the big universe and God, if there was one, to help me, as only it could.

I begged like only the desperate do. This was my last hope. I rocked on the couch, clutching my knees, and the world seemed to still as I let go of fighting for a solution to heal my soul and body. I gave way for something bigger to intervene. Or release me.

Then I fell asleep.

In the next vivid flash of Sunday, I promised Dandelion a picnic in bed. I stumbled off the couch to open the door for Gino's delivery guy. My girl was twirling on the floor next to me, happy she would soon be filling her belly with fettuccine Alfredo in a bed picnic with her mama. I was wearing only a T-shirt, panties, and bad hair, and I knew that something wasn't right. Everything trembled—hands, legs, arms, fingers, toes, torso, head—and I moved like someone or no one directed my body and my thoughts. I'd become a peculiar, half-dressed woman flinging who knows how many bills at the guy at the door. Money fluttered past his hands as I jolted the door closed. I didn't care. I couldn't.

Upstairs, Dandelion had supper in the linens, and I slept in the crust of her leftovers.

Suddenly, something with no definition, an urge of unknown origin, awakened me. I flopped out of bed as if I were an object on the ocean floor, pushed and pulled and moved by forces not my own. A haze was all I perceived. Before I reached the doorway, the urge exploded, and foreignness shot out of my mouth like missiles blasting dark blobs that landed everywhere. They kept coming. I tasted something foul. My thoughts swam like uncatchable fish, yet I grasped that this was no ordinary vomiting. This was projectile . . . shit. *This can't be good.*

My hands shook as they reached for the top drawer, where Vicodin was hidden from young curiosity. Popping half an elongated pill was an impossible action. Two or three pills, or perhaps a handful of them, fell into my mouth and onto the floor. Calling 911 didn't ever swim by. I tottered to the bathroom to brush the foulness away from my mouth and T-shirt. I pulled off my dirty underwear and reached for toothpaste. Then I felt my brow hit a cool surface.

"I hear you won't have a CAT scan."

"That's right." Sunday's snapshots scatter when Jim's double appears next to me. His voice is sonorous and pleasant. On his white coat is a name tag that clears away my confusion. "Dr. Hunter."

"You're a tough one." He doesn't argue or rattle off medical rules I won't get today. He smiles.

I like him. I like his ruddy face. "What makes you think I need one?"

"Because I say so."

That's it. That's his explanation. Dr. Hunter is a confident man, and I like that. I like much about him. "Okay," I concede. "I'll have one."

WHEN I RETURN TO the ER, Cal is still there, on the same chair, wringing his hands.

"Why are you still here?" I demand.

He fake-laughs. "Somehow, the cops got Ma and Pa's number from your cell and called them. Ma then called me. I just happened to be around." A new, post-matrimonial pause. There's no rush in either of us today. "Belle noticed the mail piling up and how the bathroom light was staying on. That's why she came to check. They're diamonds in the rough. Saints."

A faint image flashes of Jim appearing next to me on the cold tile, shaking my body, calling my name. He kept calling, even as the ambulance pulled off.

I nod. This now feels like someone else's story. Someone else is in this hospital bed. Someone else was on a floor and found by neighbors who are saints. This cannot be my story, but it is, they tell me. Another terrible place to be.

"Do you know Dandelion was dehydrated and famished when Belle got her?"

The ache for the little girl who was presented with such a big task. I can't go there. That's where true pain lies.

Cal leans over and, in a familiar whisper, he mouths, "Do you know I was interrogated for hours? By the freaking cops! And by that friggin' doc of yours. A social worker, too. It's too fucking much. I've done nothing illegal!"

"Why?"

"They thought you were a drug addict. That doc kept claiming you were. Your blood levels showed sky-high narcotics." Another fake laugh; drugs are always funny. "The asshole doc insisted those scars on your legs were cigarette burns. He wouldn't give up and insinuated Dandelion was abused. That's why the snot-nosed social worker came."

"You're kidding me." The lesions have turned to jagged red scars, ugly reminders of all that was found in Atlanta. Maybe it *is* my story. *Social Services showed up.*

"I kept telling them about Crohn's and the painkillers you've been on. I guess they finally believed me. You really need to teach her how to dial 911."

Without warning, Dr. Hunter and a clipboard show up. He's got some explaining to do. "I hear you thought I was a drug addict."

He nods but doesn't smile. "It's surprising the narcotics you ingested didn't kill you. The marks on your legs looked suspicious. In actuality, the narcotics probably saved your life, cooling you from a raging fever that would have killed you. Or caused brain damage." He stands quiet for a moment. "Look, we got the CAT scan results back. They show what I expected. You need emergency surgery."

"Why?" The question of my life.

"Basically, your intestines have ruptured. The CT doesn't show many details. The surgeon will know more once he begins operating." Dr. Hunter mislays his somber look as he adds, "You're in luck, because our best GI surgeon happens to be on call today. He'll see you shortly." He rests his hand on my shoulder. "Any questions?"

I shake my head. Aside from wondering why the nurse has strapped my right leg to the bed so I can't move it, I have no more curiosity in me today. This really cannot be my story.

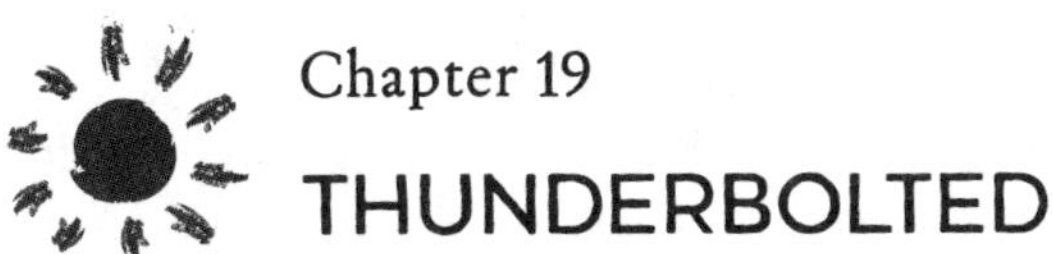

Chapter 19
THUNDERBOLTED

I am in another room when I open my eyes again. Its lights cast mellow shadows on a gray wall. Four scrubs, one white and three green, are gathered in a corner; one breaks off and walks to my bedside.

"Ms. Nilsson, I am Dr. Green. I am going to do your surgery." He doesn't shake my hand or rest his hand on my shoulder. I know he is wary of germs, and extraordinarily serious-minded.

"Hi, Dr. Green." I smile. "You don't recognize me? Must be because you're used to seeing me from behind."

The Nilsson sense of humor can feel so bad to those who aren't family. Dr. Green stares blankly at me as if Emil himself just poured blood sausage makings onto his head. Deep silence. Being a colorectal surgeon is, indeed, underrated, serious business, not something you weave into a joke with three grave surgeons next to you.

"I'm one of your patients, remember?" I remind him. "You've been monitoring my skin tags."

Maybe he has lost recall. *I* haven't forgotten the past year of submitting myself to hemorrhoid exams at his office—dropping my pants at the assistant's order and waiting with my bared buttocks on a raised platform, my face pressed into a paper-sheeted surface. Suspended while Dr. Green fastidiously latexes his hands and then does his business in my rear. So yeah, he's used to seeing me from behind. And after each exam, I've caught disagreeable grimaces flying across his face as he's removed and discarded the soiled gloves, clearly avoiding looking into my blue gaze.

Dr. Green's lack of eye contact has been the kind of thing that has ruined a whole week leading up to an appointment. If only he would stop scribbling in my file for one moment as he told me there was no malignancy and then reminded me to come back in four months. If only he would look at me.

I've long pitied Green's wife. He has a photo of her and their three children in his office. Now I am learning he is St. Mary's best surgeon, and I am lucky to be at his mercy, again.

"Oh . . . yes, Ms. Nilsson." A flash of recognition enters below the John Lennon glasses Dr. Green assuredly isn't wearing for fashion reasons. He steps forward. "Ms. Nilsson, you are very sick. I will do my best, but I am not sure exactly what I will encounter once I begin operating."

"All right," I say. "As long as I'm able to travel to Denmark for Christmas. My flight is in two weeks." I've made up with Mother Karin and need to go home to spend the first Christmas at Halfdansvej 9 without Mag. The trip is nonnegotiable.

"I am sorry." These three words turn Dr. Green into someone I haven't met before. Mostly, I hear softness when he continues, "That won't happen, Ms. Nilsson. This is serious surgery, and you won't be able to travel for a while."

"I can't have surgery, then," I say. Sudden sobs erupt. I did not foresee such an inflexible answer, even from Dr. Green. "My father just passed, and I need to be in Denmark with my family." Were it not for the leg that apparently isn't strapped but simply numb, I would throw linens aside and jump off this bed.

More softness. "You don't have a choice, Ms. Nilsson."

Now I truly hear Dr. Green, and I realize, at last, that this isn't someone else's story. It's me in this hospital bed, me who is very sick and facing a very grave situation. "How bad is it?" I press the words out.

"I *will* do my best," he says instead of directly answering my question. "I understand you have a daughter, and you need to see her before surgery."

This can't be happening. Hands find my face and rock my despair into the hospital world. I might not wake up again and see Dandelion. That's what Dr. Green is saying. Surgery may not save me, and Dandelion could end up mama-less. I might not make it. *How will she, then?*

Dr. Green doesn't leave. While the hospital linens turn damp with sorrow, he stays next to me until the new reality finally fits.

When the indelible is your enemy, and you have to move forward, acceptance can be pressed into a time tock. Sometimes, yearning to leave life and yearning to live life are just breaths apart, a faint time tock with St. Mary's best surgeon at my side.

"Thank you, Dr. Green," I say through a hiccup. There is only one way forward: I am going to get through this and still be Dandelion's mama. We're going to be together, dawn and dew, for many more years. We're going to make everything better, together.

Will is a visceral thing; right now, it is fueling every speck of me to be life, animating the former strong Viking body to do what it has to do to pull through surgery. To do what others doubt it can: live.

"There is one more thing." Dr. Green is still standing by the foot of the bed. "I will probably need to construct an ileostomy. It will be temporary."

No! The frightful thing I've suffered so long to avoid, escaping Danish docs who assured bag surgery and life quality and sticking with Doc H, who prescribes McDonald's and never a pouch operation, has just shown up in this gray room. Slender, fine-boned Dr. Green unintentionally just uppercut me.

"You promise? You promise?" I am not asking. "It won't be forever?" I am begging. Losing my life or living with a stool bag—both are unlivable options.

Pretty brown eyes look at me from behind the round spectacles. "I promise . . . it won't be forever." In solemn seconds while he speaks, the old Doctor Green disintegrates as if a cleaning maid has quickly and efficiently Windexed him away, and a tender, benevolent man takes his place—someone deeply sincere, skilled, and with great passion for his trade. I know this is a man I can trust with my life and my fears. I got will, and I got Dr. Green.

I exhale, deeply. Maybe Mrs. David Green mostly sees a husband who provides well but works way too many hours, giving his time to the OR and office patients with gastro-rectal woes. I see a doctor who sees his patient and offers her the treatment that must be part of any health-giving protocol: presence, compassion, and humanity. That is the strongest way to enter a surgery that may not be enough to save your life.

"Thank you," I whisper. My response is not a matter of form; it is filled with the original spirit of gramercy. Before me, I see a doctor who has already saved his patient.

Dr. Green wavers but doesn't step closer. "See you in a couple of hours, Ms. Nilsson. Don't forget to see your daughter."

SOMEONE CALLS BELLE, and in no time, Dandelion is on her way, her belly full from the extravaganza next door. Suddenly, her fair hair appears, uncombed and tangled, in the doorway to the gray room. My little girl doesn't rush to throw herself into my embrace, however, but instead stands stiff, as if tacked to the opening. Her dad is a silhouette behind her, and I see a new shadow in the face of my six-year-old. Dandelion doesn't know what is happening. She doesn't know why her mama didn't get up and why we are apart. Why there are dirty plates in the bed, and why the school bus doesn't get her. Her world was just thunderbolted. Thor got her, too.

I force a wide smile. I am not going to give any attention to what could be our finale, if will and Dr. Green weren't involved. I am not going to prepare myself to let go of her, or her for a mama-less future. Hurt and tears are too big to be let out; they will take everything in their path, and this hospital moment is forever too short, too precious. By choice, I am going to inhale this moment for all the life it's got—and now, at last, Dandelion is throwing herself into me, her familiar body warm against mine.

Her chatter and questions kick-start, and we are wonderfully, awfully, joined in linens that never will be anything but washed-out gray. And that's a universal favor. A break, a benediction unlike any before, and then it hits me: As I answer Dandelion's questions about the lines in my nose, the beeping machines, and the Starbucks treat of the day that Belle got her, it's as if I am embracing one of the Great Wonders of the world—inexplicably beautiful, awe-inspiring, mysterious—and gratitude strikes full force, like a special-edition universal nudge. My little girl, who is just six, never left; she stayed, being the presence of dew and daybreak that I needed to stay. *She fed me her breath. She gave life to my second chance.* When I was brought to my knees, no longer kissing the world . . .

Gratitude pushes everything aside, all the stuff my body has been catching up with. Here, joined with my daughter among lines and beeping sounds, the day is suddenly a miracle to me. She has given me the thing that shouldn't have happened but did, as if a reverse birth took place in our bathroom. All at once, it is as if the sun, the moon, and the entire star universe are stuffed into me, my own private galaxy born from the breath of a Dandelion, and I clutch my girl and feel like the most spectacularly blessed being in the world. How wonderful, how gifted I am to receive all this.

That's a formidable new presence on a very bad day before big surgery.

Dr. Green reappears. "I have just spoken to your sister in Denmark. She is on her way. She should be here when you wake up from surgery."

I stare at Dr. Green. Nothing makes sense once more.

A soft voice unravels it for me: "We honestly didn't know if you would make it when you arrived. I have been in steady contact with your mother and your sister in Denmark. They purchased a ticket straight away for your sister."

"That's great," I say. Then I realize that it *is* great. Sallie and I haven't spoken since I called the cops on her this summer. Despite everything, there's no one I'd rather leave my daughter with. Something heavy departs the gray room. Sallie will fill Dandelion's Danish Christmas calendar with loads of chocolate. I am not so alone, and thankfulness has hold of me.

All too soon, Dandelion is gone, and I am wheeled into pre-op.

A YOUNG MAN STANDING in darkness greets me. I don't know where I am. The young man bends over me, his hands busying themselves somewhere along my body.

A voice rustles: "It's leaking."

A thought sways by. *Oh.*

The young man removes something and leaves it in heaps on a table. I am trying to make sense of who, where, why, what? *Oh.* I had surgery. I look down and see a miniature

Mount Everest jutting under the blanket. Before I sway away again, I wonder what's under the white bulge where my abdomen used to be.

That's the farewell I get to give to the strong, athletic, wonderful body, honed through a childhood of unintentional parkour with the boy band. It has carried me through so much—to this room, to this night. It has been my ally, trustable above all else. Now, a male nurse is removing the dressing on a body transformed. A makeover has been forced on my ally. That's something for which I could never prepare.

A body isn't just a body, not in my world. It holds my identity, even if quotes claim, "You are not your body."

Fudge that. I am *also* my body.

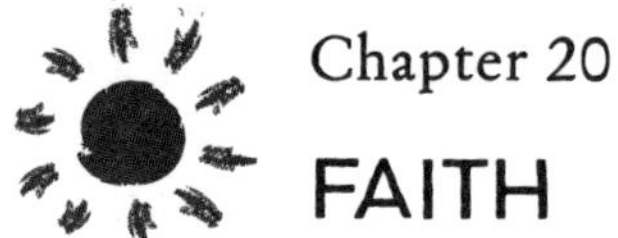

Chapter 20
FAITH

Next time I open my eyes, Sister Sallie is sitting on a chair in a corner, her brown hair tilted against another gray wall. Despite her closed eyes, I rasp, "Hi."

In no time, she's at my side, and tears, hers or mine, gush. We try hugging, but there are too many contraptions between us. Somehow, our hands find a way through hospital devices and join, clinging to one another, and this past summer and the years behind it are no more. *My sister is here. Thank goodness.*

"Oh, Nette," she weeps, and her tender hand strokes my cheek. The look on her sorrowful face takes me aback. Her hand, her face—it's all new.

"So you *do* love me." It's not a question but a surprised statement.

"Of course!" Her hiccups say it all. "*W-we-ee . . . w-were so-o . . . afraid y-oouu woul-dn't . . . maak-ke it-t.*"

Her touch stays on my cheek while I take it in. Love is a beautiful thing, even—nay, especially—in post-op surgery, when your life has been saved, and your big sister has your hand.

Two things jump out at me: First, the person I was yesterday is gone because I have just emerged from a womb; the past, the surgery, the Sunday, the coma, the incandescence, maybe all of it united. I am a newborn with gratitude. I am fresh and clean, the tarnish of old gone, wiped out. A big sense of gratitude fills this wake-up room.

Second, pain. I am in pain hell. I hurt like nothing has ever hurt before. Every speck of me is ablaze; it's as if my body exploded and burnt, charred pieces are what I am. It is a foreign, foe-like sensation. It cannot be ignored, no matter the army of IVs and poles around me. So I cry, from pain.

"I know," Sallie whispers, her touch finding its way back to my cheek.

Sallie has been through a couple of touch-and-go surgeries; her life was a question mark for three long months when her first pregnancy had her hospitalized, and premature Cody was born filled with IV morphine. She knows the role of surgical pain. This helps, a little. My big sister knows what to do, and she makes a nurse arrive with a needle full of attempted relief. When she tells me she's only staying a week—it's Christmas, and the kids need her—the go-to tool between us, wordless pouting, isn't even an option. I do need my big sister for much longer than seven days because Dr. Green was right: This was no easy surgery. But something new has gotten hold of me.

"Okay," I answer. I am alive, and anything coming my way is outright good favor and fortune, even if it means my sister is leaving too soon.

"I bought you this." Sallie hands me something from her travel bag.

Before she reaches my hands, I know her name to be Meredith, this lime-green wooden girl with hair made of yellow yarn gathered in two long pigtails and wings that match. She's whimsical and delightful, and her smile blinks formidable mischief. She isn't just any trinket or angel girl. The gear of religion isn't Lutheran or Danish or Nilsson, and I, who've barely had a doll before, have certainly never had an angel. She is perfect. I press her against my chest.

Then Sallie fastens her to the bedside table.

"Does she know I had surgery?" I ask.

Sallie knows what I'm asking. "Yes, but she can't talk to you. Dr. Green has kept her updated. It really didn't look too good, and when you finally came through . . . it was just too much for her. But she is paying for everything."

I don't say, "Of course." It matters, but doesn't, that Mother Karin didn't get on a flight with my sister.

Something shifts, and scrubs, white coats, and nurses with rambling patterns on their uniforms begin arriving. They invade the room with questions, probing, IV bag swapping, and procedures that check and re-check the patient and her equipment. Sallie leaves for my house, to nap and to hang Santa surprises on Dandelion's calendar while she's with her dad for the day.

Suddenly, a nurse's sharp voice halts everyone's ministrations. European phone calls must have some sort of rank because everybody disbands when she places a phone next to me.

"Is that you, Nette?"

I hear Mother Karin's mess of a quivering voice in the receiver, and I sob in reply. *How I needed to hear my mother's voice.*

"I've been so afraid," my mother whispers. "I . . . I . . . we thought . . . we lost you."

Now her cries are true and full—no drama, no hysteria, but heart. The heart of a mother who thought she lost someone precious. And I hear her. I hear my mother, at last.

"I sit by the phone, and every time it rings, my heart jumps with fright," she tells me. "I've been glued to it for days. Dr. Green has been so kind to me, calling me with frequent updates. Now he doesn't have to anymore. Oh, Nette . . . "

The great involuntary being of gratitude, and my mother, who thought she lost me, has me finding new ways. It has me saying things I have never said, no less entertained, before. "I love you, *Mor.*"

And the thing is, I do. It is the only way to answer the call. In this new life, the flawed, bereft, half-crazed woman who birthed me owns my affection, and in a big way—the way belonging to a mother, no matter her deficits. Because today, I don't see deficits. I see a mother who called, and her voice offers me everything I need.

Something exposed escapes across the big water.

"I love you too, Nette." My mother says it. Amid catastrophe, another wondrous first. Her words are like a warm glimmer of sunlight during a terrible calamity.

Then, I let her be a mother. I hold back no more. "I did . . . *nooot* think it'd be this *haaarrrd. Iiit* hurts *sooo muuuch. Annnd I cannn't cooome hooome for Chriiissstmaaas.*" I surrender a daughter's ache into the receiver for a mother to catch.

And she does. "I know, I know. But it'll be okay. You just focus on getting better, okay? Listen to Dr. Green, okay? You *must* listen."

"Okay." I quiver, feeling all the okayness in my mother's catch.

The transformative power of a trauma is like a fire on a parched field, a usurping force that destroys to bring better life to the body it decimated. Yesterday's daughter is gone. The stuff that wouldn't be purged before now, has been. When I reach in to feel the familiar story of betrayal and hurt, it is gone. All the old, dead stuff no longer matters, and in the gray room, in a moment alone in the washed-out sheets, I hear my mother—and love is all I find.

We hang up. For no reason other than the fact that I am alone in a hospital room and conscious, the effortless gratitude expands because I realize the perfection of the terrible thing that nearly killed me and how my life has been saved in five ways. That's a lot of perfection. In the darkest hour of my story, I bowed to the universe, and life turned sublime; it responded in no time and found a way for me to bear change, as if it had been kicking its heels, waiting for me to issue a genuine call for help. A change I never would have opted for, but now I am in its embrace.

Dandelion didn't dial 911 or run for help, the biggest save of all. She simply stayed—an unswerving little body, the sole presence that could stop me from gliding away with the incandescence. The delirium of shooting shit had me lose my exacting ways with pills, so Vicodin, known to kill, instead saved me. And when time was running out, on both the little body and the bigger body on the tile floor, the saints next door busted into our home to rescue us.

The following save and perfection, of course, was having the best GI on call the day the coma ended—and the best Dr. Green is. He got me through to waking up to see my sister, tired from traveling but at my side.

I don't know yet that having Sallie here in the hours to come will be another perfect save, and I also don't yet know that being unable to walk, unable to escape from the hospital linens, in bed with everything that needed to go, that needed to change, will prove to be yet another—perhaps a last resort in that big blueprint of mine.

Meredith, too, will get a turn to be my savior. Something is still raging, it turns out. The truth of gratitude will get another test run. So I won't forget.

I don't know when it starts, when time turns fuzzy. Suddenly, I am in the ICU, my eyes are half-open, and through the fuzziness, I get that this is not a place you want to be. Everything is intense here. The nurse doesn't leave but stays, fiddling with IV poles and riggings around my body; the door swings open with an invasion of white coats, clipboards, new orders, and bright, unremitting light that outdoes the NYC theater district at night. A new level of charred agony overwhelms me. I am no longer able to feel the big being of gratitude. I am no longer able to think of my little girl and the ache of missing her—missing *us*, as we have never been apart like this before.

Then Sallie is at my side again. She has returned from a shift with Dandelion. She tells me what's going on.

"You have to relax," her sound begs. She strokes my hair. "The doctors can't get your heart to slow down. It's in overdrive. They have tried several medications. Please . . . relax."

The smile on my sister's pretty face doesn't brighten the room. Her smile is gone. That's trouble. Because Sallie smiles through everything.

The ICU efforts with my refractory heart are like a cartoon rolling before me. I am watching the tense ministrations happening. I never think, *I'm in trouble, and they are saving me.*

Then providence, or perhaps my blueprint, sends Jimmy, the night-shift nurse. He's an older guy, someone you'd take for your mechanic, not the man checking the medical gear that's keeping you alive. He is also the first staff member to tell me why I am in intensive care.

He sits down on a chair next to me. "Sweetheart, this is critical. Your heart's racing uncontrollably. The meds aren't working. They're out of options. You have to slow it down. *You.*"

Jimmy stays sitting while his words find a way through the pain and into me. In the room's darkness, fear overwhelms me. No intense care is saving me, and I am just a handful of amok beeps from dying—that's what Jimmy is telling me. Clearly telling me. Screeching beeps on the monitor next to us chime in.

"Slow it down, honey," he whispers. "You got to." Nurse Jimmy not only speaks, but he also speaks my language—not the disconnected medical code of regular staff who don't utter much of use but in kindness, the sound that will make me listen.

I do listen. I must take this into my own hands. Jimmy is telling me it's up to me to find a way back from the edge. Big gratitude is involuntary when you awake to a second chance, but so is fear when you realize the second chance is about to pop.

I can't let this happen. I reach into the past, to the place where wound and power arise, a joint force in origin. I reach for my mother's finest moment, and I know what to do. Hands down, no doubt, I know how to divert fear and crash its course. I fix my eyes on lime-green Meredith, wings and all, and I begin praying.

Faith is my superpower, the unintentional gift Mother Karin bestowed on me one dark nighttime in the upstairs bedroom when it was I—not, for reasons that have been erased from memory, Sister Sallie—who was sleeping in the empty bed next to Mother Karin and her growing, pregnant womb. Faith is a wand that has made me believe in all things—people, chances, tomorrow, and, above all, in that big thing in the universe that holds your hand and sees you through when nothing else can.

I was nearly six, full of preciousness and the rare privilege of resting my cheek against a pillow upstairs. My mother and I were alone in the quiet dark, and like the softest of rustles telling you nature is breathing even if night obscures, I listened to the soft breath of her round body next to me. An unknown world embraced the bedroom, like nature at rest. I wasn't sleeping, and neither was Mother Karin.

"What are you doing?" I whispered.

"I am praying to God."

Her mildness from talking to God spilled into a fine whisper before her soft respirations returned. I'd known God before from the bedtime prayer, "Now I close my eyes . . ." Mother Karin had taught it to Sallie and me, a prayer passed from Mormor and through generations of mothers before her. But now I knew God for real. Mother Karin was talking to him in a way she spoke to no one, and despite her growing womb, she was so little and true, her folded hands giving away things to a benevolent being. Her finest gift for her second daughter was that she showed how faith was done; she showed how to be very little and vulnerable and trust that something bigger would guide you through. Before sleep overwhelmed the bedroom, I knew I could trust not just God but also my mother on this one. That was outright a superpower.

With two helpers next to me, Jimmy and Meredith, I invoke my superpower, and I begin praying. I pray to the lime-green emissary of the big being my mother made me trust, and I pray to survive. I pray for tomorrow. I pray for my life to be extended, to live to see the morning sun and Dandelion. I pray for my second chance to stay. For hours, with my eyes fastened to Meredith and her look of mischief, I pray. An intense desire is all that I am, despite the pain hell and beeping monitors, and my prayers run through the night.

When you choose faith over fear and leave room for nothing else, fear must retract. And it does. In the wee hours of a new morning, I slide into sleep.

WHEN I WAKE UP, Jimmy is gone, and Sallie sits in the seat. I am still alive.

Sallie's eyes are hazier than ever. "You *have to* relax, Nette," she says.

It turns out it isn't over yet. Stuck in the washed-out linens of a too-bright room and fogged with drugs and agony, it would be easy to give in and let faith slip away. Thank goodness it's December. Faith is a gift that keeps giving, if you let it.

"Can you get me the radio control?" I rasp through the fogginess.

Sallie hands me a device with dials and a tiny square for a speaker. Her eyes express inquiry.

"Find a station that plays Christmas music," I say.

In seconds, the soothing notes of John Lennon enter the room, and I press my ear against the control to "Happy Xmas" and the music of a war that is over. Next comes "Glory to

God in the Highest" and "Rudolph the Red-Nosed Reindeer." Carols, jingles, psalms, and holiday music of all sorts stream into me, and I attempt humming along to the spirit of the season as it streams into my ear. For hours, I ignore my sister and everyone coming and going through the door. I ignore everything but the balm of Christmas music. On and off, I slide into sleep, but as soon as my eyes open, I reach for the tiny speaker again.

That is how you survive another day of ICU when it is on you to slow down a heart gone berserk. You locate the spirit of whatever sustains you in whatever way you can, be it a mischievous-looking angel, Christmas music, or anything else.

Though my heart and the beeping monitor have slowed down, even faith turns out to be inadequate. My lungs have started giving in, and severe respiratory distress in tandem with a freezing kind of survival terror has entered the bright room. My brain suddenly can't move. At that moment, when the radio ceases to soothe me, and I can't think of a prayer to send up—that is when compassion carries me through to another morning sun.

Once again, I have no idea when or how it starts. Abruptly, I am behind a black mask that covers my entire face. I have lost the ability to respire; I gasp, but nothing enters. I am choking in the panic of not getting enough air.

Mercifully, the black mask oxygenates me.

The doctors don't know what is causing the respiratory distress and have issued several tests, Sallie tells me. She has returned from another shift at the precise time when I must have the mask removed, and for long seconds live the terror of exposing myself without the fake air support.

While the black mask is my protector, it is also my prison. It feeds me life, but wearing it makes me feel as if I am standing with my face against a forceful fan blowing continuous, chilling, killing air, with no option of running away. The airflow is so strong that matter gathers in my mouth—dryness, hair balls, phlegm, and other tiny, unidentifiable objects—as if the fan is pulling everything out of the room's atmosphere and impelling it into my mouth. Every few hours, the collection becomes insufferable, and it must be removed—and for seventy-three fretful seconds, I snap for air, already feeling the crush of death moving in before the nurse has even pulled out a swab.

The nurse takes too much time handing me the swab. In rasps, I beg her to move faster.

"You'll be all right," she shoots back and turns around to fiddle with something, then steps to the sink. She needs to hand me the black mask, and it's not coming. I am gasping, like stranded bait left beached by careless fishermen. I am dying.

Just before I do, the nurse brings the protector, and I throw it back on for another false breath.

The next cleaning is merely another replay with a different nurse. I will be all right, she says, too. I don't feel all right. Hysteria grows like a Mother Karin bush behind the mask, and I can't sleep or find any soft spot in the graying linens behind the protector. I can only think of the next time I must face a nurse and the too-slow assault of the swab.

A new angel is at hand: my sister. As if it's her life vocation, Sallie slides into the original meaning of the word "nurse," and she gets me through the daytime. We communicate using hand signals because the black mask stops me from speaking. She brings a little blue notebook from the local pharmacy, purchased so I can spell my needs and worries in it. She has no trouble receiving my messages, and in no time, we make an exact science of mouth-cleaning. She lines tools up for me—water, basin, swabs, wipes—and in supported seconds, I rid my mouth of the room's garbage. A simple thing and not a dreaded assault, if you listen, not to mention a detail that alleviates purgatory for this particular patient.

Something unnamed in the ICU stops the nurses from honoring these directions, no matter my writings and no matter Sallie's verbal requests and sticky notes, and terror shows up every night when the mask must be removed, absent my sister's attendance. Unable to protest aloud, I must endure the nightly swab asphyxiation assault.

Other things I must endure also. I learn so after going to the MRI room without my sister trailing the bed downstairs. Sallie is tirelessly driving up and down the Boulevard, taking care of both sister and niece, and sometimes I am left on my own in the big world of the hospital. The doctor crew shares a predilection for MRIs. Barely a day passes without a visit to the dark basement for a check on my heart and lungs. My big sister is my voice; knowing my terror, she digs out firmness from below her goofiness and uses it to make clear, precise instructions to the staff. The trouble is that the black mask must be left in the ICU when we go down for scans, and a tiny white tube, attached to a portable oxygen tank, becomes my temporary air supplier. It's a very poor substitute. To make matters worse, the tube must be surrendered during the long minutes when I am lifted onto the MRI bed and the whirring machine above me captures what the doctors need. Sallie makes the nurse assigned to minister the oxygen equipment promise to listen to me. The nurse pledges to stop the scan and give me a thin flow of oxygen if I ask for it. So simple, isn't it?

But today, Sallie isn't present when it is MRI time. I plead not to go downstairs. My voice adds up to nothing.

I know I am in trouble when the bed reaches the elevator. "Yes, of course," the nurse answers, yet she barely glimpses at my directions in the blue notebook. She's young and chatty, and she and the aide are striking up a smiley conversation. My notebook doesn't exist. Neither do I, it seems, because the nurse removes the tube while looking at the two male technicians in the MRI room, not at her patient. She doesn't catch the fluttering of my eyes seeking hers. The mask is off, but I can't speak.

Inside the scanning machine, the terrible air hunger digs into me. *I am dying.* I try to scream, but that doesn't work either. Before the whirring is complete, one of the technicians turns rescuer. He orders the nurse to bring the oxygen tube fast.

Upstairs, the on-duty nurse notices my incapacitated state and calls for new instructions from a white coat. Everything in me feels plundered, and not from loss of air alone. The doctor orders rest and no MRIs for a few days.

Surviving the ICU is really about so much more than a bad set of heart and lungs. *Where would I be if Sallie wasn't my voice?*

ONE LATE MORNING, my sister shows up and asks, "How are you?" Then she commences her daily bulletin of my little girl, who's staying overnight with Belle and Jim, eating dinners with other friends, and carrying her nightgown around just in case Sallie can't come home for bedtime. "Dandelion's wondering why her visit with you was canceled—"

Hurried words in the little notebook interrupt her. I cannot answer or listen. Not today. The mask doesn't allow for crying. Seventy-three seconds, let alone seventy-three hours, is insufficient for the kind of tears stored behind the black mask. They can't be allowed to escape, both because of the mask and my desire to survive this overly bright room.

They are always there, but today, there's one more reason for my tears.

Business starts at dawn in the big hospital, and a little while ago, I found my face covered in sterile dressing while two white coats leaned over me. One of them was about to make an incision in my left carotid artery, I gathered from their exchange. My neck was twisted into an abnormal stretch while a rough hand applied suffocating pressure on the dressing area. I had no voice and no body to signal my distress.

"Why don't you put her on a respirator?" an accented male voice asked. The knife cut my skin. "That'd be so much easier."

He was talking about me. A patient. In his care. He might as well have stated, "Why not put her down?" Same rate of care. Same indifference. Same attack while some sort of tube got inserted into me by two white coats who never spoke my name or saw my face below the blue dressing.

Being on a respirator is awful business, but worse business is being perpetrated by those supposed and paid to make you well. Rape has many shades, and the shade in the ICU this morning got me good. To them, I am prey in a bed, not a patient.

Why don't they care?

It would be so easy to dip into the mad river of anger—hate, even—again.

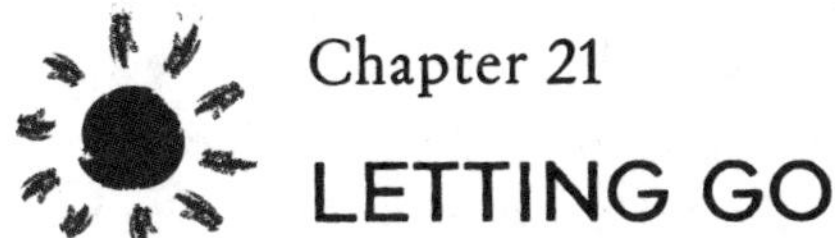

Chapter 21

LETTING GO

I do make it out of the ICU. I am in step-down, a room with an intermediate level of care, because my lungs and heart are no longer failing. The mask is gone, and the notebook is no longer on the table next to me. Both are small signs of improvement.

When Sallie shows up late in the morning today, I've been dreading her arrival. The look in her hazy blue eyes tells me she, too, is fighting this day. She takes my hand and stands next to me. We both half smile and let silence speak our ruefulness.

"It's okay," I finally squeak.

Sallie's suitcase stands by the door. A cab is on the way. In two hours, she will be at Newark Liberty International Airport for her return flight to Denmark. "The kids need you. You . . . have . . . I wouldn't have made . . ." I don't finish the sentence. I can't.

My sister is one of the few people who knows my scent as well as I do. That's unavoidable given that we, in a long stretch of early childhood at Friggsvej, shared a bed with wide, fluffy pillows in the gut of a dark basement those nights Magnum was home, and in the dark space before sleep arrived also exchanged pranks and secrets. I was never afraid of the dark, because I had my older sister next to me when the lights were out in the big room. Despite our challenges over the years, only my sister could have carried me through this past week, past the darkness. She knows nearly every corner of me, and she too has fought to stay alive from a hospital bed, with her young child in someone else's care. With steadfast love, she knew intuitively how to guide me through. No space is wide enough to hold my gratitude for her, for what she has done, and for the unexpected strength of our bond. And now she must go.

If I speak my sorrow, my heart will surely crack.

Sallie squeezes my hand. I sense mounting tears behind her eyelids. She sniffles and pauses for a moment. Perhaps she is sensing a clock ticking somewhere, because she pops an unexpected question: "Do you think Dad had other women?"

I look at her. Then I smile. Widely. Broadly. The hospital world around us fades. We are two sisters sharing in a way only two Nilsson sisters can. Sharing a family piece that has marred us and our upbringing. My relief is palpable, and I chuckle. "You know!"

Sallie isn't smiling yet. Her look is inquiring. "What did you find in the apartment? You found something, didn't you?"

And I tell her everything. I tell her about the contents of Magnum's desk drawer, our inheritance waiting for someone to show up and claim it. I tell her about Magda, the stack of photos revealing a love affair with Czechoslovakia for twenty-some years, the little girl with Sallie's same broad forehead, the address and phone number listed over and over, the scorecard . . . all of it comes out.

The shocked look on Sallie's face is so brief it barely registers. She, too, is chuckling now. We are both letting go, of a childhood and years where Czechoslovakia played a role that we couldn't put a name to but left us with an uneasiness that we tucked away, that we never shared. We do now.

"Remember the crystal glasses he brought home, the good ones saved for special occasions?" Sallie recalls. "He was so proud of them. Maybe she picked them out for us."

I do remember the wineglasses and tumblers with delicate, handmade patterns cut in crystal glass. Mother Karin, always wearing a grim-faced expression, laid them out next to heirloom silverware on a starched white tablecloth for special events like Christmas and Easter.

Sallie and I both crack up at her joke. We share the same brand of humor, and in a wordless exchange of understanding, we laugh uncontrollably at the paradoxical fact that Magda resembles a dark version of a younger Mother Karin. A fact that is stupefying and yet heartwarming.

Everything is falling into place. Pieces that didn't fit anywhere now have a home, and our shared laughter lets the confusion and lie of the past leave. We don't think to blame Magnum. I have already come to terms with his misdeeds, and we have, each in our own way, moved past unforgiveness.

Time presses against us, and Sallie is, for once, full of questions. "You still have the photos? I want to see them. You really think the girl is our sister?"

I answer every question, and as I do a new softness, just in time for my sister's leaving, moves into me. I am no longer alone in this unbearable situation. I am no longer the keeper of the family secret—because it is no longer a secret. My sister has made sure. She has torn the dark family lie open with her questions, asking for revelation. Once again, she has come to my rescue and helped me when I couldn't do what I needed to do. She is my sister, in the truest sense of the lovely word.

"And Mother Karin?" she continues. "Does she know? She probably does."

I relay how Mother Karin does in her own way know about the real role of Czechoslovakia in Magnum's life, and in her own way doesn't want to hear or see the details. Right or wrong, neither one of us wants to force the truth upon her.

Sallie leaves. The sorrow I feel at her departing, knowing we won't ever again experience the intimacy that only life's most vulnerable times bring on, is quickly replaced with a new and surprising state. My body can let go now—of everything it has amassed and held on to for years, of the stockpile of pain the shocking discovery in Atlanta only added to—because when secrets are shared and acknowledged, they lose their power.

It is about time.

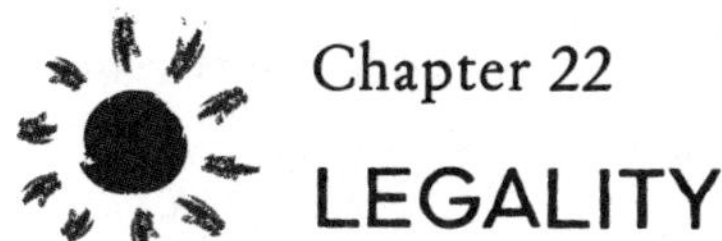

Chapter 22
LEGALITY

Though Sallie is gone, my gratitude for everything she has done sticks around. Her last deed was to arrange for more family to come to me and to Dandelion at the house. Aunt Margit and her youngest daughter, Rikke, are on their way to cover the stretch from Christmas to New Year's. I am not alone. People are coming out of the woodwork—calling, visiting, sending cards, flowers, trinkets, and prayers, and offering services of all sorts. The story of Nette on a bathroom floor, her daughter next to her for days, and the touch-and-gos in the hospital is a wildfire that brings out the best in everybody who hears of it. They all want to do good and, truly, in this pre-Facebook era, I didn't know I had this many friends or that this many people cared about me. Talk about a gratitude generator; it's so grand it could charge the entirety of St. Mary's.

It's been exactly eleven days that I haven't seen Dandelion. Each day in the hospital has deepened the drought in the spot inside of which my girl alone has dominion. Aunt Margit and Rikke have just brought her to 307, my new room.

My heart beats wildly when I see her. She looks different. Her six-year-old smile is gone. Standing in the doorway, she bites her nails, though there's little left to bite off. She hesitates and clearly doesn't know how to enter.

From the bed, I tell her Rikke and Aunt Margit will be staying at the house with her. Her eyes, the color of moist soil, finally light up at the sound of my voice, and in a flash she takes her spot in the bed and leans into me.

Cute, twentysomething Rikke has the gift of being naturally adorable, and kids love her. Dandelion is no exception. But her glee is short-lived. "Mama, when are you coming home?" She pauses. "The princesses are very sad. They miss you. Ariel misses you most."

I stroke Dandelion's silky hair and wish I could stroke her nails back. Those ragged, almost-gone nails on those little, innocent fingers. It is awful seeing my girl this way. I lengthen the short moment; then I must speak.

"You've been such an amazing strong girl, sweet pea. I'm so proud of you. But I need for you to be strong a little while longer. It's going to take the doctors some time to help me get better. Perhaps you can let Ariel and her friends know I'm coming home as soon as possible?" It takes all the might I have in me to speak and not crumble.

Against the hospital gown, Dandelion murmurs, "Daddy says I have to go to another school."

"What!" My body tenses.

"He says you have to stay here for a very long time, and I have to go to school in Florida with my cousins."

"Oh, *skattepige*, that's just a silly thing your dad's saying. I promise you won't have to change schools."

This promise flows easily. I have always made each and every decision when it comes to our little girl. Busted intestines and a long-projected recovery time don't change the fact that I am her only true parent, whereas her dad is an unpredictable visitor without a schedule or commitment. Of course she will be staying in Seaside, in the routines and the school she knows. Mrs. Roe, her teacher, is an extraordinary mothership who provides such care and predictability for her students that she's already a second mother to my girl. Of all times, familiar structure is critical to Dandelion's well-being right now, as is the short drive down the Boulevard to St. Mary's. We've never been more than a few night kisses apart, and splitting us up now would be an outright absurdity. Another trauma like an out-of-state move is the last thing this child needs. Dandelion must be embraced by the place she knows as home in the weeks ahead. Children are fragile beings. One blow and—poof—they're gone.

OVERNIGHT, IT SEEMS, I have become a seventy-five-pounds-overweight freak, adding new water bulk by the hour. My body can't keep up with the continual orders for more IV fluid, and my tissue is so stretched that I suddenly have serious curves. I am beyond uncomfortable, and the medical vacuum cleaner roving my abdomen, where surgery has left a gaping hole that must be cleaned of fluids, only adds to the distress. The daily dressing change when a young doctor checks on the hole and the hospital Hoover is also a dread to endure. I don't want to witness the atrocity below the mound.

The three drains hanging off my body in various positions are harder to ignore. These containers for various body waste tend to find their way into my new rolls and curves. To boot, my numb leg has been diagnosed with severe neuropathy, meaning the nerves in my leg, foot, and toes are destroyed from lying on a floor in the same position for days.

I can't move. I can't stand, walk, or get out of bed. I am an invalid Michelin Man, bogged down with devices. A crane lifts me out of bed every morning, sending my body swinging in the air, while five aides dash around me. My body and various medical gear all have to make it to the chair in one go.

Getting out of bed has become a loud, disruptive event, in the room and on the floor. Aides squeal directions and warnings, tubes and attachments tangle, and moans and sobs erupt from me because my body simply can't twist any longer. It has lost all its sanctity. It's just a thing to be handled. I wear a fluffy gown designed for openness, and the gown reveals everything, no filter. My unwashed hair is an orb of itchy bristles around my head. Who cares? I don't know—I do, but can't.

Room 307 is one sure way to learn how humiliation feels, one sure way to let go of all attachments to my body. Orders are orders, and at St. Mary's, patients must get out of bed, move their limbs, and sit up. That's how healing and discharge happen, even if it takes a crane and everyone knowing the real size of your arse.

I am a freak now—or rather, again. This condition is simply an old matter surfacing in a new way. Being this off is nearly second nature to me. Young Mother Karin decided shortly after giving birth to a child she didn't want, especially since I wasn't a boy, that I must be an ape; that was such a wacko thing to say, be, and live by, yet felt true to me because the woman who fed me felt that way. The white Afro that grew out of my head as a baby put clouds in my childhood because strangers loved to ogle my peculiar aberrant hair—and that makes Room 307 feel not at all unfamiliar.

Being a freak won't get me, though. I already know how to dodge being the aberration others watch and discuss. Besides, Aunt Margit and Rikke are taking up where my sister left off, and they bring Dandelion in for a visit every day. Sharing daily moments with my daughter—feeling her smell, her voice, her gnawed little nails—carries me through the freakishness from one day to the next. This, not the crane, is the surest, fastest way to healing and discharge. She is wonderful, and I get to hug her.

And then I don't. At the time when it matters most, the hospital or the world won't let me be a mother anymore. For days, ever since Dandelion told me of her dad's intentions to move her to Florida, I have repeatedly talked to Cal, a lawyer, a hospital social worker, and Dandelion's teacher, Mrs. Roe. But everyone agrees—Cal will get his way. There's no way around it. In the hospital, legality supersedes compassion in everything. The divorce agreement he drew up is solid: We share joint custody of our child. Even though I've pleaded with him to move into my house as a temporary solution, even though he isn't restrained by a job or any commitment, despite my and the social worker's pleas, despite Mrs. Roe's professional opinion and the next-door saints' advice—he refuses. And the others abide by his decision. Dandelion is going to Florida to stay with his sister, Theresa, and her husband and two daughters. They live an hour away from Cal's new residence in a marina in Miami Beach, and he has finagled a kindergarten spot for Dandelion in a public school in their town.

So, two days before Christmas, I have to break my promise to Dandelion and tell her she *is* going away.

I have to do all of this on the phone. She is at her grandparents' house in New Jersey and won't come by again. In three days, she will be in Florida in a new life.

I can't imagine how my girl feels when her mother turns into someone she doesn't know: a big, fat liar. She is mostly silent during this conversation.

On this awful day, being a hospital patient strips me of a human right—the right to have my daughter next to me. In this place, this human right is overruled by being locked in a bed in 307, giving free rein to an unmerciful father. I don't know how I am going to survive freakishness and everything else when my girl is gone. *What has my girl been stripped of?*

That doesn't matter to the hospital. Compassion doesn't fit in here.

Two days before Christmas, catastrophe overwhelms Room 307.

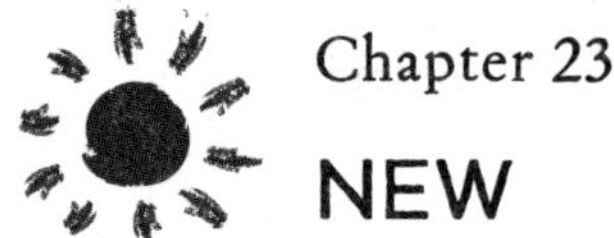

Chapter 23
NEW

My family has left, and no one else is coming. Dandelion is away in Florida, and everyone knows I know how to take care of myself.

I will need every whit of energy I possess to make it through this big hospital and into a world where Dandelion's voice isn't a fleeting thing on the phone because she's making chocolate cake with cousin Bessie and can't talk. I reach for my ancestral gift: the Viking stamina my young legs honed up a merciless hill, because making it up without collapsing, dropping newspapers, or plain giving up demanded a singular focus with no other thought allowed.

I don't cry. Tears won't help. I stay fighting and numb—that's what will get me out of here—and I take the bad days one at a time.

They tend to start the same way. Before dawn, when a wintry suit of night still blankets my window, a maroon uniform enters. With one hand, she carries a blood-sampling kit; with the other, she flips on a harsh ceiling light, waking me up. She logs another round of incessant sticks to my veins before turning off the inclement bulb. Darkness beckons, but before I can drift off, another uniform, a different color, flicks on the switch. More intrusions follow: gatherings of crucial medical data, temperature, blood pressure, and pulse. No one speaks while the task is performed—there's just a lot of frowning. The standard of care focuses on the body, not the heart.

Outside Room 307, the hallway rouses with the bustling of shift change—a medley of voices, rolling wheels, quick steps, and the clicking of closing binders sweeps into my bunk. Morning and a tray arrive, followed by two aides who strip off my linens and gown and push the detested washcloth over my shivering body, around the dressed-up hole, and into every crevice with swift force. It's a drill, and they must stay on time. I moan as they swing my nakedness into another position without any soft skill. Except my favorites; they practice gentleness when they, in their Island lilt, say, "Fuck time" and run the tap until steaming water fills the pink basin, turning the washcloth into a toasty caress, and follow my guidance.

After my sheets are changed, the nurse checks in, followed by a surge of MDs. More arrivals, scheduled and unscheduled; another tray; perhaps an in-house pastor or an overseas call; a visitor; a snooze here and there; uniforms that gather more medical data; and the crane and freaky wagon. One tray later, and then suddenly it's night, and another day has passed without tears. The day is just a check in someone's calendar.

One bad day closer to seeing Dandelion again.

AFTER AUNT MARGIT AND Rikke leave, while the bad days of January roll by, the saints next door, Jim and Belle, are with me in Room 307. Although our socks have never shared a laundry basket, our toothbrushes never touched, and we've never had adjoining bedrooms, they are with me, consoling and comforting me. Being here is not too much for them. We've become family. The couple, nearly Mother Karin's age, grew up in low-income housing in the Bronx, and a deep sense of community was instilled there because that's how they and everyone else survived bad days and hardship of all sorts. They're used to family being something other than shared DNA.

Besides, their Melissa is a fine girl a decade older than mine, and they can't imagine that blessing being ripped or shipped away. But it can happen—they've just witnessed it—and maybe that's the true reason why Jim and Belle transform into two people who do everything that the best of family would do for me in Room 307. They give everything they've got. On those days when others would leave or not show up or simply not get what's going on, they stay. Though their world is beckoning them, they stay, because that's what I need.

TODAY IS AN AWFUL day in Room 307, and it starts when the maroon uniform flicks on the switch. I open my eyes but only see darkness. I can't possibly make it through three trays to nighttime and sleep. Because today, I can't stay numb or fight. The ache for Dandelion is too terrible. I am all sobs and wetness before the maroon uniform even touches my arm. Her frown deepens, and my wails explode into the awful morning.

They continue as more uniforms and hospital schedules log in, and trays come and go. I turn red-faced and swollen, a lamenting, howling disturbance on the floor.

This is the awful day Jim walks into. He arrives directly from work, though a pork dinner is waiting at home. He's undone the tie on his CEO suit.

"Bad day, huh?" He skips his usual greeting and states the uncomfortable obvious.

"*Nooo iiit's aaawwwfuuulll . . .*" I bawl. "*Aaannnd theee docs juuussst waaannnaaa giiive meee a pppilll . . .*"

"What's going on?" Jim places his very tall figure on a chair next to the bed and folds his hands together.

"*Theeyy telll me I'mmm depresseeed. I'm not fuuucking depresssed!*" I let out a loud sob.

Jim listens while my wails continue.

"*I dooon't waaant anotheerr pilll. I dooon't waaant a shuuut-uupp pilll. A pilll for haaaving emotiiions . . . Aaam I nooot allooowed to feeel? Aaall theeey waaannt is too giiive me piiills . . . waaahhh . . . fooor deepressionnn.*"

My grief won't be silenced, and Jim listens on.

"*Theeey wannnt to curreee my emotionsss.*"

Or cover the disturbance, stop it with any drug, just have it be gone. Each time a uniform has walked through the door since my first wail early this morning, a pink pill has been offered, handed, coaxed, or insisted upon. It sits like a little devil in a medicine cup on the bedside table. Waiting to silence. Waiting to bring convenience.

"Oh Jim, *I missss her sooo muuuch.*" Then I fall apart into the pillow because I can no longer handle the changing nature of the calls to my little girl down south. There's no more glee on the line, only a thin, wan, unknown voice who cries that cousin Brittany doesn't share and that she hates it there. Dandelion's aunt and family are surely making their best efforts to embrace her, yet as of yesterday, my daughter has turned into someone who pleads in faint, inaudible whispers when I call, "Please, please, Mama, can I come home? I'm frozen like a statue. *Please.*"

In turn, I hang up before a sorrow great enough to make the universe kneel can explode into the receiver and frighten my six-year-old even more.

This six-year-old has lost all things familiar—even her mama, who always tries to make everything right with a kiss, a hug, or a few words. That's an unimaginable loss. And now she is losing her ability to cope with her new, mama-less world because I can't help her. I, too, am a wan, impotent voice, and this adds to the fright of the bereft girl in Florida. I only have more uncertainty to offer my girl. "Not yet, *skattepige*," is all I have to say and all I don't want to say. "Yes, you can," is the only right answer, but I am a body in a bed, and her homecoming is no longer within my power to promise. Legality over compassion, remember?

"Of course you're hurting. I can't imagine what I'd do if I couldn't see Missy for this long. I wouldn't have enough tears for it." Jim unfolds his hands.

That's it. That's all it takes. An acknowledgment, a caring body next to me folding and unfolding hands, and like that my awful day starts to get undone.

I grab a tissue. Hiccups have replaced wails. "*Ohhh, Jim, when will I seee herrr aaagainnn?* When?"

"I don't know, Nette," he says gently. "All I know is that she *will* come home. You will see her again. It'll take some time, but you will."

It's past 8:00 p.m., and as Jim heads home to Belle and his cold pork chop, it's not too late for another welcome presence to walk through the door. He does most other days, awful or not. He, too, has seen it all, and though he still addresses me with hospital formality, the brown eyes behind the spectacles have grown softer and even kinder.

"Ms. Nilsson is, understandably, in pain," he barks at the staff today. "Her daughter is gone. Let her be. No more antidepressants."

Most days, I mark time until Dr. Green's unhurried presence has checked into Room 307 and asked for a status update on the day's pains and symptoms. His long, sculpted hands move with care against my skin, changing a drain or checking the atrocity below the mound, and he listens as I enumerate the pangs of a very bad mattress and a nauseatingly sugary hospital tray.

Orders follow in the hallway. I overhear him demanding that a special mattress and special tray be brought to me and for labs to be postponed until after 7:00 a.m. each day. His voice speaks with the self-assurance of a brand that knows its own worth.

When vanity—indeed, in vanity there is hope—beseeches me, and I cannot help but ask about the future look of the uneven suture track from my sternum to the pelvic bone, Dr. Green's answer is unruffled, sincere: "Let's see after it's healed. We'll have Dr. Bouras give his opinion on what can be done."

I can't walk. I can't eat. I live on a pain pump, and my pupils are wide like teacups. I am a mess in a bad hospital gown—and yet Dr. Green takes my question seriously, and the moment he does, I no longer feel like a body, an inconvenience, but a patient-person.

After filing orders in the hallway at the nurses' station, Dr. Green makes a second appearance in my room to give a status update on my new compression boots.

Dr. Green is an exceptional doctor in a place that seems less intent on healing wounds unless it coincides with business and protocol, and can be charted. He may be a surgeon, and a fine one, but he is also a holistic practitioner—at least in Room 307 he is. He intuits that wounds require much more than a knife and a drain to heal. He *always* lets me know when someone else will be covering his rounds the next day. He is someone a patient-person needs more of, not less.

He helps me transform.

While January rolls on, gratitude sticks around. It overrules the leg pain, the misdeeds of frowning uniforms, and the hole in my soul from missing my girl. With Dr. Green, I have a whole lot to be grateful for, and that's not going away. *Thank you, Dr. Green.*

A new body but also a new way. Maybe that's the real healing I'm undergoing at St. Mary's.

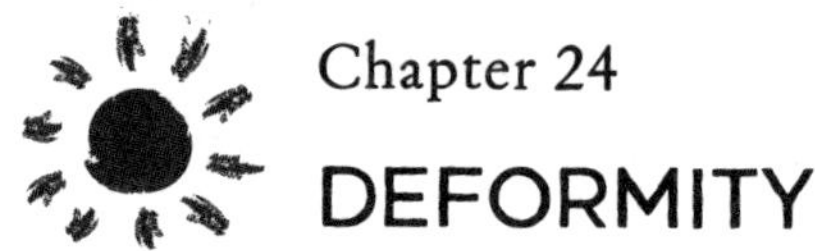

Chapter 24
DEFORMITY

"We could get a bigger pair." Abby stands with the biggest shoe that can be had in her hand. It's an aqua-colored sneaker. Her specialty, aside from being a woman architect resolving structural building issues all over the city, is helping others. She's also my neighbor, to my great fortune. She's been shoe hunting on my behalf and has brought me three pairs of jumbo sneakers.

"It's no use," I whimper from the linens. No one, even Dr. Green, can help the tortured foot. Nerve pain has its own category, and I keep pushing the morphine pump to little avail. My foot is bigger than a size 12, much bigger than the aqua sneaker that really isn't a sneaker but a ship. It resembles the giant metal hulls resting on the piers of Frederikshavn, waiting to be turned into fully operating container ships. I didn't know they made shoes this big. Yet the sneaker ship isn't big enough. My former size 9 is a limb my brain no longer can direct. Its only response is shooting, burning nerve throes that only intensify when Abby tries to squeeze it into a jumbo sneaker.

These days, in late January 2006, three aides are next to me when I wobble off the crane and onto a path of cushions leading to the armchair. My right foot feels as if it is burnt char, and I need shoes to tolerate standing. I need shoes to make it away from the crane and out of the room with a walker. Yet it won't work. The foot is too swollen, and it is too excruciating to wear anything but synthetic hospital socks. And it's not getting better.

"I'll find some bigger ones, men's size. That should work." Abby gathers up boxes. She knows the world always has a solution.

I want my neighbor to leave. The room is suddenly too small for her kindness and persistence. This capsized attempt to wear the sneaker ships she brought me is a wake-up call. I am nowhere near walking.

I don't even know if I will ever walk again. No one tells me anything. No one tells me if my foot will restructure itself, build itself anew. Or what to wear. It's as if there's a big blemish in this room, just like in my family. The foot has been sent downstairs for innumerable CTs and tested and charted, but where are the white coats with a prognosis? Where is the protocol when you really need it? My foot is a body part preferably avoided by those in charge; its true state is hidden somewhere in a test result or chart. When I ask for a foot forecast or a footwear solution, all I get is another stack of hospital socks and silence. There is a great, big quiescence in Room 307 that doesn't serve the patient.

Even so, I must make it work. I need to relearn how to walk, not knowing if my foot will ever have that capability.

I watch Abby leave. There's no humor in me today, and not just because of the sneaker shipwreck, but also because I hear the freaky wagon creaking down the hallway. Talk about a real cover-up. Mary pushes the dreaded wagon around the big hospital, offering her services to patients. She makes nice so well. Everything about her sweet, flawless face, good clothes, and mild demeanor is flowing, attractive, and inviting. Until you know what she offers and what you can't refuse. Then you turn your head and pretend she and her services don't exist.

At least I do.

Mary peddles how to confront your disfigurement for real while feigning that it's not a repugnant, soul-robbing experience to have the turd purse on your abdomen changed and see a red piece of intestine jutting out of a hole in your stomach for the first or seventy-eighth time. Mary's the crap lady—the specialty nurse called when Ms. Nilsson springs a leak. This happens quite frequently when you defecate through a plastic bag. Each time, Mary smiles and doesn't crinkle her nose at the putrid stench. She asks if I want to try, as if she's offering a cocktail at the open-air bar on a cruise ship's top deck.

Hell no!

Mary's own disgust might be silenced, but mine is so strong and sad that it is altogether gone. It is too big to live. That's why, when Mary does her thing, I close my eyes and make believe that the bag on my right side hasn't stolen a big piece of my soul. But it has. Having a plastic piece attached to my body for fake defecation is a deal-breaker, a soul-breaker. A thing I cannot accept, let alone endure. Sister Sallie's ostomy has taught me the greedy need for wipes, appliances, and running water when a leak leaves you covered in shit and people around you turn stone-faced from the stench and abnormality. Having a bag is unnatural and unutterably restrictive, and though I've never made it to the rainforest before, my soul aches from the loss of the squat-and-relieve method.

Today or any other time, I *really* don't want to look at the freakishness. I want to ignore it forever. But the little girl who wants to come home but can't removes all choice in the matter. I have to look and learn to be my own maintenance crew. I cannot afford more failure. So today, when Mary starts fiddling on my torso and asks her standard question, I finally answer, "Okay."

The ostomy nurse doesn't flinch. "Let me show you, then." She is still smiling.

I am not breathing. In seconds, when Mary peels off a square adhesive, I will be facing my deformity for real. Although my eyes are fixed on her French-manicured hands, my eyes are not seeing. That is called leaving your body—your spirit heads out, away—and it can happen when life gets beyond uncomfortable and unbearable.

It's a hole, a horrible cavity I was not born with. That's all I remember about the first glance at my freakishness.

Mary cuts and pastes away, her hands working rapidly, but her face stays calm, unfazed by the urgency of her movements. A volley of instructions accompanies her labor. "Wafer . . . your size . . . quarter-inch . . . convex or flat . . . skin barrier . . . odor control . . . good seal . . . last seven days."

I hear but don't hear her. A pile of waste is building. On the bedside table, it's as if an overflowing makeup counter at Macy's has made a sudden appearance. The brand names aren't Lancôme and Dior products in pretty little boxes, however, but rather oddity tubes, bottles, wrappings, belts, clamps, and other gizmos that Mary selects, opens, and applies in rapid, precise moves.

Still, even her extreme speed isn't enough. A gurgling sound breaks into the room, followed by an eruption from the hole in my abdomen. Fluid—*excrement, to make it clear*—shoots out, bursts into the air and lands . . . everywhere. This is no leak but a volcanic eruption, a freakish occurrence, and it soils linens, gown, bed, and everything but Mary's hands. Her artwork is destroyed.

The stench is one that no one can flee. And the extent to which it soils my soul cannot be told.

Mary beams. "This can happen. You'll learn to work fast, but we do need to start over."

Room 307 is a cartoon now, something I am watching from afar with my eyes shut.

"Do you want to start emptying by yourself?" Mary is filling the garbage in the corner. Her artwork is seemingly done.

Several times a day, an aide armed with a plastic bottle enters the room, steps up to my bed, shoves my gown aside, unclamps the pouch, and sticks the bag opening into the bottle—all while frowning a great bit—and then squeezes the pouch like someone milking a cow. It takes skill to get everything out while avoiding a spill-out and linen change. My chart is marked with the mL content of each offloading for whoever takes an interest in my current stool tally. Everything about this intervention feels as if someone's using my body against my will.

I don't know how I answer; all I hear is the specialty nurse responding, "All right, see you soon."

I watch her leave, ready to push the squeaky wagon on to the next pitiful soul.

My deformity is worse than anything I ever could have imagined. No one ever wishes to be a miscreation, and I no longer have a way to handle mine. I feel so bleak now, knowing the truth of the disgust that I am. Yet there is a brightness in the bleakness that cannot be undimmed or taken away. I am one step closer to seeing my girl of dew, and that day cannot come soon enough.

While the sound of the squeaky wagon fades down the hallway, I am thinking of Dr. Green and the lifeline he has given me. He has done the finest thing a doctor can do when it comes to my new warped body: He's given me hope.

I recall opening my eyes in post-surgery murkiness and seeing Dr. Green's face and tired, benevolent eyes before me. He was explaining the long surgery I had just survived: ". . . and the ileostomy is only temporary, Ms. Nilsson."

If I could have moved, his hand would have been in mine, tightly squeezed. "You promise, Dr. Green? Really, you promise it's only temporary?" I pleaded through the murkiness.

"Yes, Ms. Nilsson," he assured me. "It is only to give your intestines a rest. When you are ready, we will reverse it."

The deformity is only short-term. My GI tract will be restored, suited to rainforest survival—and that is why, apart from saving a life, Dr. Green has done the finest thing a doctor can do. Other doctors might have handled the same situation in a hundred different ways. Dr. Green knows to speak to that which will help me get past the unacceptable.

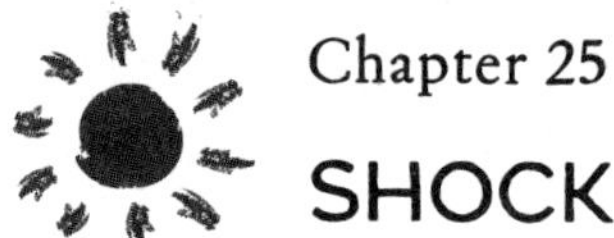

Chapter 25
SHOCK

The first tray has been delivered, and the TV blasts sound into the room while I wait for the cold basin and a uniform to arrive. I am expecting this day to be just like any other.

"Good morning, I'm Caroline. I'm here to discuss discharge plans with you." She looks like an elf—petite and perky, too well-dressed for a hospital wage, and a clipboard rests in her hand. Elves can be very tricky.

"Excuse me?"

The elf lady speaks as if I know all about the kerfuffle she's bringing into Room 307 on an early February day. "I'm beginning to look into rehab options and want to go over a few things with you." She clicks her pen in fast, short chinks.

I say nothing. Rehab is a universe I have no concept of. It is not something a thirty-six-year-old thinks of, even when she finds herself waking up after a coma with a crippled limb and a stool bag. When it comes to this word, rehab for the rich and famous is all I know, and that is universes away from what the elf lady has in mind.

"Now that you're taking a few steps, we can't keep you. Maybe we can get you into a rehab facility." The elf lady makes a rapid check on her clipboard. She's been doing this for years, clearly, because she knows where the check must fall without even looking.

My eyes are growing wider than teacup size. "Huh?" is all I manage.

The elf lady loosens her grip on the pen and steps to the bedside. Her face softens, and the next check on the clipboard is ignored. Already, I know she's someone's grandmother, the kind who adores all her offspring.

"Insurance companies aren't easy to deal with," she says. "But I heard your story, and I'll try to get a good facility for you."

"I'm not going home!?" I cry out. I am too confounded to ask: "What are the not-good facilities?"

"Oh honey . . . no, you're not. But the insurance company wants you discharged."

With the support of a pair of hands, I am just making it to the armchair in my synthetic socks. I assumed this bunk in the big hospital world would be my life until better times arrived. Given my socialist upbringing, I actually assumed more: that St. Mary's would choose the best, not the most cost-effective, option for the patient. I receive an abrupt lesson in American capitalism as I realize this hospital will discharge someone who still can't reach all corners of her crooked, aching body with a washcloth, someone who can't get to a toilet bowl independently. This hospital will abandon a patient to whatever place her pocket covers—even if that simply means "out the door"—rather than ensure she goes to where her healing needs will be met.

"What . . . what is . . . is . . . a rehab going to do for me?" I stutter, though what I want is to throw myself under the linens.

"They have a much better PT department than we do," Caroline says. "It's in your best interest to go to a place where you can concentrate on getting on your feet. That is, if I can get you in somewhere. I have yet to figure out what your insurance will cover. In a week or two, I hope to have you placed." She shakes her silver-hued pixie cut and smiles as if she's just brought me the best news in the world.

A week! Inside 307, I know the dreaded morning wash routine, the icy basement, and its MRI machine, as well as how to reach the call button. Who knows what kind of washcloth, basement, or buzzer awaits me in rehab?

This morning, a kerfuffle has landed in my room, and I don't know how to breathe through it—because, suddenly, I don't want to meet my future.

"THAT'S GREAT. Can you do one more?"

Another step, and the big armchair is behind me, out of sight. Slowly, attentively, I peg my entire consciousness on raising my right foot before lowering it onto the slippery hospital floor. The foot smacks against the pale gray linoleum all at once, as if I am a puppeteer who has lost control of the wire to the figure below. My hands clutch the walker, and I shift my balance to move my left foot. This step feels nearly normal.

Today's PT session is special. I lift the right foot again. It hits the floor like a dropped plate crashing. I can't answer the young uniform; a throat bubble obstructs all speech.

"Do you need to rest?" The nimble uniform who moves with an athlete's grace, like I used to, is behind me, rolling the IV pole, her hands poised for a body catch. She's unaware of how dear her agility is.

The allotted twenty minutes are up. I nod.

Everything in me aches with faintness. My gait is like crashing plates; I'd fall to the ground without the walker, and a set of PT hands is needed for accident backup—yet today is my inaugural day of walking, of gaining back a memory after being tied up in a coma and to a hospital Hoover and towers of medical equipment for two months. It never once crossed my thirty-six-year-old mind that I could lose the faculty of standing, of putting one foot in front of the other. Until I did. Today, I am taking the first steps away from the armchair to gain back what may be possible.

I return to the washed-out sheets, and I give way to the throat bubble. It is pure joy. The joy of victory. I feel as if I am resting in the most luxurious bed, alive with the grandness of living, for I have just earned something so valuable that even the most opulent, five-star hotel stay would be no matching prize.

Then exhaustion gives way to sleep.

THE NEXT DAY, the nimble PT is back, and once again, I direct my feet past the chair. The door opening is like another hilltop, and I have plans to make it through today.

"Of course, I'll do one more," I answer the young uniform. The Viking stamina isn't lost. It'll be the last thing ever to go.

"Nette, you're doing great!" A familiar voice appears. Caroline, without her clipboard, steps up in front of the walker. A smile settles on her face. "How many?"

Chelsea answers for me: "We're up to five today."

"You're definitely ready," Caroline says. "Subacute, I'd say. See you tomorrow. Maybe I'll have news for you."

I don't want any discharge news, though I do want to know what subacute means. This word has no comforting sound. Yet there is no room for questions. When Caroline makes her daily appearance on the third floor, all my attention is focused on taking steps in the hallway, or I am enervated from walker walking. So Caroline does all the talking.

She could stay in her cubicle somewhere in this big place and guide the rehab approval process from there. Instead, she takes the elevator, presses 3, and shows up every day to deliver a personal announcement of each new step, along with personal tidbits about her attorney husband, golf dates, and big crowd of fabulous grandchildren. She informs me that she's looking at several facilities and that "subacute" is the right fit. This type of facility offers intense PT—two to three hours per day in a gym-like atmosphere, but with medical staff. She has determined that I will be best served by a local, reputable facility with a younger population. Caroline is crossing many extra *T*'s in this particular rehab clearance; she has even sought out additional recommendations from colleagues in other hospitals.

Caroline is no longer the elf lady but someone who makes up for annoyed, callous nurses in a rush, doctors who see a consult and not a person, aides with no finesse, and other uncharitable uniforms who add to the discomfort and angst of living in a hospital bunk. Small acts of kindness are treasures when you're confined to a room where even a glass of water is beyond your reach. When you depend on uniforms for all your needs, you quickly learn how to tell a person's true character because they can make or break your day—and night. When you've been ignored, forgotten, dismissed, bypassed, huffed and puffed at, and treated like work or a thing that must fit into a schedule or someone's whims, small acts of kindness have an exponential effect—they are like seeds in a bleak desert that immediately blossom into beautiful, gorgeous, balmy flowers. I dare not think what type of facility I'd be dumped at if Caroline were one of the huffing and puffing, annoyed uniforms that see a chart and not a human being in Room 307.

I am blessed because Caroline has turned into someone whose rehab judgment I trust all the way.

MORE THAN A WEEK moves by. The walker and I are down the hallway. Chelsea is several feet behind us with the IV pole. The clattering sound of scurrying heels makes me slow down, and I can't miss that Caroline's feisty sparkle is amiss, her eyes signaling alarm.

She pelts a question even before reaching us: "How many steps are you putting down?"

"Ms. Nilsson is doing real well," Chelsea sings back. "Around eighty."

"Good." Caroline slows to a walk. She looks at me, no giggles today, and states, "We really need to get you out of here. No more than eighty feet, okay?"

Wait! What? It turns out that too much success, too many steps in a hospital hallway, can be a really bad thing. Each day, the walker and I are getting farther down the hallway, passing more doors—and we shouldn't. PT is a game, a calculated numbers game played against the other players, insurance companies and facilities, who are required to approve a patient for subacute care. Too few or too many steps will disqualify the candidate. PT uniforms must play along with game rules and stop me in my tracks before I pass the hundred-foot mark, or at least indicate in their notes that I've ambulated less than a hundred feet but more than ten feet, or else I will be denied subacute care. No SAR—subacute rehabilitation—will take me if I can't shuffle at least ten feet, and the insurance company will deny coverage if the walker and I can manage a hundred. Eighty seems to be a safe number. Caroline is just a cog holding the game together, and though she doesn't intend her visit this morning to feel like an ambush, an ambush it is.

And it doesn't stop there.

I am leaning on the walker, not daring another step as long as Caroline is on the floor.

She continues the rules sneak-attack. "Honey, Glen Crest has a daily co-pay. Are you able to cover it? If you need to stay longer than twenty-eight days, insurance won't cover it. Can you handle self-pay cost?"

What's she saying? Twenty-eight days! The cost is immaterial to me, but the time is not. Time is all that matters to me. I need time with my girl. Being out of time is something that neither she nor I can take much more of. Now I am learning I am more than twenty-eight days away from wrapping her into me.

The hallway air abruptly turns oppressive, like I'm wearing another black mask; only the walker keeps me from falling onto the floor in a crying, bewildered, dumbfounded, sad mess. *It can't be twenty-eight days. Or longer! Please, it can't be.*

How long does it take to learn how to walk? How did twenty-eight become a magic number? My body has lost all flexibility, and yet it is being ordered to bend and fold according to rules that don't have its recovery in mind. My needs are unimportant; only the needs of the insurance companies are being tended to at this critical juncture. So, yes, I want to fill the hospital hallway with wails, not just for my girl down south but because the medical system that supervises my care and recovery is one big, awful game, structured to abandon the patient and overrule her healing concerns when doing so serves its economic interest—which is most of the time.

My grudge—this day, when Caroline turns out to be a cog, and for years to come—is the misrepresentation the big hospital system deploys. St. Mary's claims to be one of the nation's leading cardiac care programs, yet it upholds another cover story. For all its "care programs," I've yet to see any true caring endeavor in this place. In fact, truth seems dangerous here. Truth will put a patient like me on the curb on my disabled feet, unless I am lucky enough to get staff assigned to me who are so kind that they'll play this big game on my behalf—stretching notes, looking the other way, stopping me from succeeding too much, or even lying on my behalf. I don't want to go away for twenty-eight days, and I object to having no say in my treatment plans, but desperate as I am, I know that to let myself be discarded by the medical system, left on my own with the new, fragile body and the accoutrements I don't yet know how to care for, would be an outright unsound idea.

If you ask me, the real disease is not in the patient-person but in the medical system itself. Perhaps the medical system, too, burst somewhere in its adulthood and was sewn together all faulty and flawed, disease its new way. Ruptured at its core, corrupted. Because on this day, when Chelsea finagles her notes to get me into a reputable SAR, it is blindingly clear to me that the hospital has lost its way from a blueprint that outlines an honorable, admirable intention: We care.

Hell no, you don't.

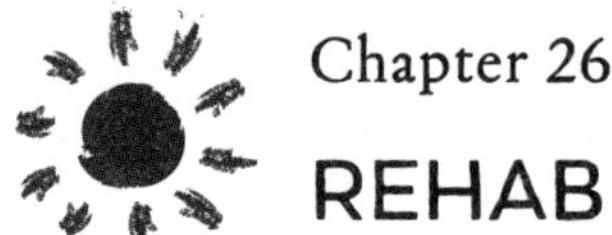

Chapter 26
REHAB

I am tied down on a gurney, straps around my arms and legs. The ambulance bumps along a private, tree-lined driveway; glimpses of winter-barren branches enter through the tiny square window in the transporter. Glen Crest approved my admittance just yesterday. I am the right amount of disabled for this SAR. The EMT sings out that we're almost there, but that doesn't stop the fluttering of my heart. I am very nervous about what awaits me at this new care facility.

The large Gold Coast property I'll be staying at overlooks the Sound, the water that also surrounds our home on Long Island. Only the very privileged get to behold it from their bedrooms, and soon, I will be one of them. Caroline has made sure.

The big estate the ambulance is driving toward was built with oil money for an industrial baron decades ago. Both the Gilded Era and the baron are long gone, and the big limestone structure with a slate roof and imported European marble has found another purpose: rehabilitation facility.

The ambulance bypasses the main entrance's grand black gates and pulls around to a basement door in the building's rear. The gurney, the straps, and I are soon rolled through a set of double brown doors.

I blink. A long, narrow hallway with weary-looking, mustard-green walls stretches out before me. Stark light from ceiling bulbs reveals linoleum flooring of a nameless color, though blotches and stains create their own kind of unkempt pattern. There's no gild here, or graceful aging. A smell I can't identify smacks against my nostrils. Winter-fresh scent never reaches these halls, it also tells me. The former Gold Coast basement entrance makes St. Mary's seem like a true five-star resort.

The glass pane in front of a small cubicle slides open. Three rotund women sit behind it.

The most senior and most rotund speaks through it: "Hannah will get you a wheelchair while I do the paperwork."

It must be me, on the gurney, she's addressing. I may be thirty-six years old, but I might as well be a toddler with no familiar hand to hold on to, for lonely and lost is all I am in this ugly basement where gilded privilege is but a fake promise.

Before I know it, I am sitting in a wheelchair, hugging the bag of belongings from home Belle packed for me, and Hannah, the cubicle's youngest, is pushing me down the mustard-green hallway.

"PT will show you how to operate the wheelchair," she prattles. "I think it might be Sean Sean."

I'm wheelchair material. I clutch the bag even tighter. *What happened?* My soul doesn't go for being bold or brave, not anymore. It reads danger signals like others read *Newsday*—first thing in the morning. Entering a rehab facility dressed up in a gilded facade with a physical body out of order and heading down a hideous hallway in a wheelchair spells peril. Too much peril for comfort. So far, Glen Crest is providing no reason to want to stay.

"We're going to the second floor. You're so lucky. Sean Sean is great. He'll be your regular PT." Hannah presses the elevator button while her chatter swirls around us. I'm hardly listening. "Do you know if you need OT? Lucky you. You got Glen Crest's only single room. Caroline insisted you get your own room. All other rooms have two patients."

Outside the elevator, Hannah waves in her sweet way. "Hi, Matthew."

Wisps of silver on a bony man in a wheelchair roll past us into the elevator. Striped PJ pants reveal gaunt ankles in a pair of slippers as unkempt as the linoleum floor.

"*E-ooo.*" A droopy mouth spits out Matthew's greeting. Although the right side of the old man's body slumps, a knotted left hand maneuvers his wheels past us.

Hannah bends over and leans into my ear with a whisper: "Stroke."

I'm still not listening because I am looking at the broad corridor outside the elevator and its sad, fatigued seventies trimming. The corridor is dorm-like, with one door after another occupying either side. Many of them are open.

"Hello, Mrs. Soretto. How are you today?" Once more, Hannah leans her whisper into me—"Diabetic. Bad one." She pushes me past the woman, who's using one leg to navigate her chair forward. There is no other leg. I am without sound.

Although the broad corridor has generous room, it seems cramped. I spy endless sets of nighties and shabby robes, messy hair, and unshaven elderly faces. I spy no pretty penny but instead a flock of wheelchairs crowding the long hallway. I spy, I spy . . . *Oh no!* This is a cosmos apart from the game I played with Dandelion. I spy no tennis racket but instead a hallway of people gone to pot—infirm, decrepit, defective, enfeebled, and scruffy. Most are geriatric and in wheels; missing body parts abound. I spy sadness, gloom, lethargy, misery. And odor. The nameless, odoriferous smell that hit my nostrils downstairs acquires an identity. It's a foul brew of unwashed, ungroomed, decaying bodies quartered inside a dwelling where fresh air isn't permitted. A noxious and stale mélange of personal smells at their nastiest. Whiffs of industrial cleaning agents don't cover it up.

The foul brew conjures up the poorhouse in Lonneberga, where a penurious collective—tattered, destitute, useless, and unwanted cast-offs from society—bunked while waiting for the Angel of Death. A sad, sad bunch. That no one, even Emil, could save.

I want out of here—immediately. This place is worse than the big hospital I just left. "This is it: 212." Hannah stops next to a piece of paper taped in a hit-or-miss manner on a door. They've misspelled my name, in crooked letters. "You're home."

What happened? Did a Royal Caribbean ad ensnare Caroline?

"You're so lucky to have your own room," Hannah repeats as we enter. "Only thing, you have to share a bathroom with next door." She points to the closed toilet door inside my new home. "No worries. They're in diapers. Dementia. Bad ones."

Room 212 has weary olive-green walls, a cot-like bed with metal rails, a rotary dial phone on an unsteady bedside table, a dresser with dark, chipped veneer, and a clunky TV screen straight from the seventies. The room is a mockery of its opulent mansion past. A barren place, long overdue for a revamp. I don't feel lucky, no matter how many times Hannah insists I should. There are at least three things I want to do: scream, pound the walls, and call Caroline on the rotary to give her a piece of my mind—*This is not up to snuff!* But I am too dumbfounded.

"Bye, Ms. Nilsson. Sean Sean or someone from PT will come by."

The door closes, and I am alone in the weary olive-green room. In a wheelchair. I don't move. My brain, too, has stopped all motion. I just sit there. Time ticks away while I remain a silhouette in the middle of ghastly 212.

The weight of my bag from home cuts into my legs, causing my brain and senses to return. I don't know about my soul. *It's just twenty-eight days. I'll see her in twenty-eight days. I can do it. I must. Must.*

The window begs my attention. I need to see the blue home beyond the fake mansion.

First, I need to make the wheels move in the direction I want. The rim on both wheels has its own unique layer of filth, its metal sheen incognito. I want a rag and soap, but I don't see a call button anywhere. Despite my resistance to touching the filth, I can't stay stuck. My hands reach down to grab the rim, and I learn being a wheelie user isn't simple. I fumble for long minutes just to make the short distance to the window.

Clank, clank—I pull the string, and dusty louvers dance aside to reveal the world outside. Gray, leftover film from years of wet weather streaks the pane, but the vista is unmistakable. I've got a panoramic view of the black tar of a parking lot complemented by several huge, snow-covered dumpsters in one corner. There is no blue; there is no green, even. There is no privilege. There is only black tar that never makes it into any advertisement. Its real story is way worse than the big world of the hospital, and I am stuck, truly stuck, in it. Neither my legs nor my wheels will allow my fleeing.

I am angry, I am sad, and I really need to pee. I need a bathroom. Now. Mere hours ago, a St. Mary uniform removed the catheter, and I haven't been on a toilet seat in months. I need help . . . but none is coming.

Down south is a little yellow flower who succors me and stops me from breaking down and giving up.

I wrangle the wheelchair to the door, which I wangle open. "*Hellooo*," I call into the corridor.

A bag of bones in a robe inches his way past 212, clinging to the bar mounted along the wall. He doesn't flinch and creeps on without pause, as if deaf.

Down the hallway, I spy no uniforms, only more tattered robes on wheels.

Then, magically, a pink-uniformed woman walks by with a rapid stride. "Someone's coming." Her impatient voice lingers behind as she disappears into the place that is long past cure. I shut the door as quickly as I can, trying to close out the Angel of Death that's hovering so conspicuously out there. I am a freak among freaks. *One of them.*

The door won't close on the notion that I am still a freak, the boy-girl with an Afro like Diana Ross's. In the north in the seventies, a white Afro was a deviance. Hair like this didn't fit any known mold and was quietly considered an abomination of nature. Each time young Nette showed up somewhere, neighbors and the world beyond stared at the anomaly, as they would now. *One of them. Someone others gawk at, but no one misses.*

Wrath is a powerful thing. It pushes back hard against the horror of being transplanted to a wheelchair and dumped in a twenty-first-century poorhouse, with no way of leaving and no help to relieve a basic need. Wrath has no mercy on the shortage of mercy in a place of subacute care. Wrath makes this freak refuse disenfranchisement, refuse being a forgotten disabled body in a concealed prison. This time, wrath is different from the past because it doesn't hole up inside and stay silent or jump out in angry, unjust shouts. It digs its heels in to find formidability in this contemporary poorhouse no one knows about. That's a change, a beautiful change, even if I am still a freak. Because not all wrath is unjustified; some is righteous.

Before the afternoon passes, I am on a wooden, peach-colored toilet seat from another era. All by myself.

Wrath and will are powerful things.

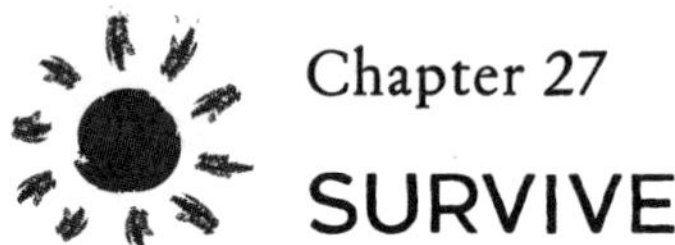

Chapter 27
SURVIVE

I'm not sure if Sean Sean is all there. He looks off—definite oddball material. A short while ago, his raspy voice called out from 212's doorway, "Ms. Nilsson, I need to show you how to operate the wheelchair."

The gangly young man with hockey-puck glasses, an old-man mustache, and limbs too big for his frame is with me downstairs. In a PT space, yes, but not the privileged place where Caroline promised I'd be doing intense physical therapy. We are in a big basement room with a few equipment stations, three whispering therapists, and three sad robes. There is no music, no pump, no drive. But the light isn't harsh and inhospitable, and Sean Sean has me wheeling up and down the floor, and doing easy turns during this sprinkling of allotted PT minutes.

"Sugar, let me take you to your room. You're doing good with your wheelchair. I'm not used to someone picking up this quickly. Tomorrow, you can come down by yourself."

Sean Sean has only been out of college for a spell, and while he has some experience with geriatric feet, he has none with a bum foot like mine. But he showed up in 212 when no one else did, and there's no one I'd rather have teach me how to walk again.

We reach the crowded hallway upstairs, and there's suddenly room for the spirit of inquiry, the extra organ that resides in me but has been turned off for a long while. "Do all these people get rehab?" I ask Sean Sean in a low voice.

Sean Sean looks cross-eyed at me, very willing to chat. "No, most of our residents don't get PT or OT. Glen Crest is primarily a skilled nursing facility, and the subacute part is a much smaller part. Very small, to be honest. You are the oddity."

A straight, honest answer at last. "You mean it's a nursing home?"

"Yes," he says, "we have mostly Medicare and Medicaid residents who require long-term nursing care. Who are not PT candidates."

We've reached 212's open door, and Sean Sean makes an unskillful wave with his oversized hand. "Okey-doke, sugar, see you tomorrow, 10:00 a.m. and 2:00 p.m. on the dottie."

I watch Sean Sean head in the other direction. He has just confirmed that Glen Crest is nothing but a dumping ground for society's poor and unwanted—those too old or broken to be fixed or those waiting for the final twitch. It is now official: Despite all of Caroline's checking, I've been placed among the dumped in a Superfund site, in a facility whose gild is in name only; Medicare and Medicaid pay solely for bare necessities. On the splendid North Shore of Long Island is a hidden storage site for freaks and the unwanted, billeted by the government, and I am in it.

I close my eyes to the corridor and its wretchedness. Like others do. I won't make twenty-eight days if the spectacle outside gets a foot in the door of 212.

SOME INJUSTICES HAVE pure killing power. For this and other reasons, the twice-daily twenty minutes in the PT space downstairs becomes a point I cling to, a brief escape from 212 and its setting. Sean Sean makes it easy as pie. In our first real PT session on my second day—twenty-six to go—he secures the Velcro on clunky weights, museum pieces from another era, around my ankles. He tells me slow and easy lifts do it, and that by tomorrow, I am going to be moving with a walker and, by the time I leave, a cane.

Sean Sean has a plan, and he has nothing but confidence in his plan—and though he doesn't know it, he is all the hope I've got. He just confirmed that I will walk again. *Yes!* If twenty minutes weren't all too short, the wetness in my chest would be let loose in the downstairs room, and I'd jump out of the wheelchair to hug this fine young man so tightly he'd cry, too. But no second can be wasted here, so instead I just nod and lift on.

Even so, the PT space has challenges. One is a full-size, wide mirror hanging on one wall. In it, for the first time in months, I see my own body's reflection. If I didn't know who I was on a hot Fourth of July in 2000, before I went soul-seeking, I am not sure I do now, in 2006. My Viking frame has turned into a stick figure—hunched, emaciated, unkempt, and aged. I am a frail body that screams bad health and no beauty. *I have lost so much . . . so much*, the mirror tells me. Muscle, strength, nerves, function, motion, youth—my looks are all gone away, awry. I don't know what or how much will return. I am a piece of scrap, a new, crippled body with nothing but deficits.

I close my eyes to the ugliness in the mirror; my reflection is a challenge I don't have room for in the days left to me here. Though my new reflection is foreign, ugly, and wretched, it's what I've got. And I actually hold gratitude for this bag of bones. It's what will allow me to walk home.

First, I need shoes, Sean Sean tells me. If I don't get shoes for support and stability, I won't get walking. The large stock of polyester patient footwear from St. Mary is grievously holding me back. A solution can be found, he says, even for an oversized foot like mine. But I must get it myself. In this place, you may be crippled, not walking, on wheels, missing body parts, and yet it's on you to procure the things you need.

At this point in time, internet shopping is not yet a reality, and the closest solution to my problem can be found in a specialty shoe store miles away. Glen Crest is located in a secluded area so off the main roads few people want to visit the facility, and I rarely receive visitors. Only because a considerate friend agrees to drive me to the store am I able to get shoes for my walking training.

Do others in the corridor need to go to the specialty store? *How does Matthew get the things he needs?*

I end up with a pair of blue sneakers that fit my giant foot—an outright blessing. In no time, I am in the hallway, hugging the wall bar like the deaf robe-wearer upstairs, each step an excoriating adventure. My body is learning the art of walking anew, all on its own, but this time, scars, tissue, and nerves are resisting, and pain meds become a comrade to get maximum steps out of PT. My two daily twenty-minute sessions are all too brief, with no allowance for additional drills, even though I want more.

On weekends, with Sean Sean and the other staff at home, the downstairs is a dark space—barricaded, as if a big storm is expected. For two days of missed PT opportunities, I hide from the scourge of the corridor while waiting for twenty minutes on Monday, and nothing has ever seemed a longer wait. Though rehab is a challenge, I welcome it like nothing else. Rehab is both an escape from the gruesome poorhouse and the road to the final exit.

OTHER TORMENTS CANNOT be escaped at Glen Crest. I'm staring at a cold tray. It, too, arrives three times a day, the same as at St. Mary's. Though this tray is no sugar overload, but mush. Always, brown mush. Most of the things on the plate in front of me on the wobbly bedside table cannot be assigned a name; they're innards of various cans that have been microwaved to a disgusting brown pulp, one ingredient resembling the next—peas 'n carrots, mashed potatoes, pseudo gravy, same heap of brown. There's not a single piece of fresh, live food. No raw victuals, no salad, no ripe fruit—not even canned, oversweet peaches are available. I've asked. The uniform answered, "Not possible. Have someone bring you fruit or veggies if you want them." Her eyes seemed to say, *Why bother? The afflicted in the hallway can't chew anyway.*

Maybe that's why what we get here at Glen Crest is chow most people wouldn't hazard to feed their dog. Mormor always had a stocked victuals storage room in the basement on Friggsvej 6, and I grew up with everything plucked from the abundance of the season and turned into homemade food, a natural way that I've tried to live by after my child entered the world.

I try again, but the brown mush just won't go down. It sticks in my throat. The tray is outright an abomination. It nourishes no one.

I am lonely, and I am famished, and food is another thing I must procure on my own at Glen Crest. I can get apples, bananas, and other perishables when my kind friend Karla answers the phone and finds time to shop and drive through Long Island traffic and sleet. She brings several real meals the first time—crunchy green vegetables tucked into rice next to moist chicken thighs. But the uniforms catch on in no time and declare it against site policy to store patient food in the floor's only refrigerator. I cannot find a way around the uncompromising storage rule, and begging my friend or a rare visitor for policy-approved apples, crackers, and bananas only feeds me for a couple of days, if rationed well. I've been robbed of so much, and now I am also being robbed of the opportunity to support and heal my body through the nature-provided tool that nutrition is.

What we feed our bodies matters. Especially when we are healing, as I am now. Wholesome nutrition really is rather simple. Mormor's recipe still works: Good, clean, local, seasonal, fresh food brings balance. The brown pulp and the daily supply of four candy bars from the vending machine downstairs, which I've resorted to in an attempt to quench my ravenousness, do the opposite. This sugar explosion is not what my body needs. But needs are not welcomed at Glen Crest. Aside from a cot and a few PT sessions, what I can't get for myself, I must go without or suffer its absence. This facility requires residents to be mechanical beings—moving, crawling, wheeling through the corridors, not needing anything, just barely breathing. This SAR is a place to survive, not a place to heal.

Here, uniforms only make scheduled appearances to bring pills and mush, and the misplaced call button is a useless piece of scrap that never gets you anything. Not even a pink apparition peeking through the open door to ask what you need. Which is why now, more than ever before, I am left on my own with the bag. Lying in a St. Mary's bed with an appliance attached to me bears no comparison to wearing one here at this Superfund site. It is a truce compared to war. I am learning that having a shit bag is so much more than high-maintenance when you're out of bed and wheeling and no uniform arrives to help you unload. I have become an overworked plumber who must get the hang of unscheduled leaks without supervision or advice from experienced staff.

And leaks tend to happen more often than not, no matter what I am doing—leg lifts, wheeling downstairs for candy bars, or sitting in 212. The bag has its own mind; it swells with gas and nasty, runny stool like a burst-ready balloon, and it is my business alone now. Daytime leaks I make it through; it's the code brown at night that's the trouble. When a smelly dike alarm sounds—at one, two, four in the morning, at any and all times—letting me know that the attachment on my abdomen has busted or is about to do so, spraying brown all around the cot and room, I need to move fast, but my movement is like pushing a ship made for ocean water across an uneven, waterless linoleum. This undertaking takes time, fumbling in the dark into a wheelchair, making it across to the cramped bathroom and onto an unstable toilet seat. I can't yet stand to unload the bag—recommended standard procedure—and so I must open the pouch's bottom closure between my legs while sitting down. That never has a pretty outcome. The released putrefaction splashes everywhere but into the bowl. And the tight bathroom is understocked, more like a latrine than a lavatory, equipped with a bare-bones supply of soap, water, and one towel, neither within easy reach of an achy wheelchair user just cut open weeks ago.

While I remain seated, holding the dripping appliance with one hand, the other overreaches to get soap to wash up the shitty mess that I am. This stretching makes the bag drip in new places, soiling more spots. Breezy toilet visits and God-given mobility are underrated, underappreciated capabilities, I've learned at Glen Crest.

I aim to make it through these code browns and all the other stuff I must get, forego, and bear. No food, no bag support, no shoe assistance, no company, and no caring won't be what kills me at Glen Crest. I've past experience with not having needs; it's like spending time in a crawl space you know of but don't care to revisit unless necessity forces you. I can—must—survive these twenty-eight days in the crawl space of Glen Crest. My little girl is waiting for me.

I HAVE MADE IT TO A Friday afternoon in late February. The date of exit is in sight. And the unscrupulousness of the fake-gilded SAR has reached new levels. I am in a crawl space so tight that each time tock has all of me enveloped in it. I must go somewhere so as not to see, feel, or acknowledge what is going on inside 212 just now. I am sitting in the wheelchair in the middle of the room, motionless like a marooned piece of Lego. Yesterday, I was outfitted with the last available skin wafer—necessary for attaching the bag—I had in my possession. For an entire week, I've warned staff of an impending shortage of supply specific to my hole, yet there's been no restocking. There has been no care to reorder. The code brown overnight and the acidic liquid that had the pouch burst at 4:36 a.m. destroyed the last wafer. There are no more. But there are sheets, a head uniform informs me.

"Hi, how are you, Nette?"

A familiar, cheery voice makes an unexpected entry into 212. A visitor has arrived at last.

"What are you doing? What's going on?" Frowns perforate Abby's impeccable makeup as she approaches the room's center.

"Hi, Abby—nice of you to come," I lie. I couldn't think of a worse day for my neighbor to show up. I don't want her here, not now. *Not like this.* Rape wants no witnesses.

Abby isn't all smiles today. "Why are you wrapped in sheets?" she questions as if I'm Alyssa, her child, not her ill-equipped neighbor.

This isn't just a bad reception. It is hands down the most humiliating moment of my life. I am huddled up in a blanket with extra sheet fortifications wrapped around my midriff where the hole is. I laugh, so I don't have to cry. "Can't you smell it? I'm an open sewer. I'm out of supplies, and the sheets soak up the runny stool my body spits out. I have to change every hour or so. Nurse's order."

Abby's nose perforce crinkles up. I can't blame her. A rotten, noxious fume saturates the room. It is way, *way* worse than the stench in the corridor because a gut rot has been let out, boosted by a candy bar overload. It sticks to everything, especially nostrils.

"It's just a little smelly." Abby is forever kind and downplays the crushing stink around us. "They must have *some* supplies. They cannot let you sit like that." She's also not the indignant kind, except just now.

I invoke a feeble, battle-worn smile. "They will." I don't have it in me to tell my neighbor that I have already asked, pleaded, begged, even threatened nurses and the floor manager to get more supplies. But there will be none until Monday—the best-case scenario. Because there are no scruples in this place. *That* account has no shortages. I am rigged up in washed-out sheets, smelling like the nastiest, most overflowing outhouse in the Western Hemisphere, and my skin is turning red and inflamed in places where the acidic sewer sauce leaves a burning trail. What's more, I am unable to stand up and change the soiled sheets as needed; my tottering balance forbids it. Fresh sheet fortification occurs solely at the mercy of a uniform visit.

And this is the day Abby has decided to visit. Her visit could have been a singular good moment at Glen Crest. Today, it is not. This moment only brings more afflictions, more degradation.

But Abby is a solution-maker. Not for nothing does she head large, successful construction projects on some of Manhattan's most exclusive real estate, climbing scaffolds and forcing timelines and city rules to be heeded despite the ensemble of building obstructions coming her way. She's used to getting—making—her way, not with her curves and chestnut Polish complexion but with sheer resolve and persuasion.

"This isn't right," she proclaims. "I'm going to talk to them."

My friend shifts into work gear, her face showing that a significant bump on the timeline at Glen Crest needs fixing. I don't say anything as she shoots out the door. I already know the outcome. Abby's efforts will be futile.

Indeed, Abby does finally meet her match today—not in the city's cutthroat construction environment, where every dime, second, and client counts, but on the North Shore of Long Island in an off-the-road human debris storage facility. She, too, must accept defeat. The uniforms, regular and head, won't extend any effort, any calls, anything, to get supplies today. Nor will they attempt to refit other sizes. Every possible solution is shut down in the corridor.

Back in my room, Abby is no longer Abby. Her tone is incredulous and shaken, and she looks like a human question mark. For once, she doesn't know how to make a situation better; all her offerings have been in vain. That's as foreign to her as American apple pie is to sharks in the Pacific. "They can't let you sit like this—it's not right," she repeats. "It isn't right!"

My neighbor is spared the knowing that Glen Crest isn't a place that does right but a place that only does wrong. A merciless place where things go terribly wrong, and no one cares. I don't want her to know. My shame is too grand even for the kindest, best-intended neighbor to bear witness. Because not every rape is a raucous assault; sometimes rape is silent, and its perpetrators are frigid, sullen, covertly aggressive people who are just making a paycheck. Pink uniforms too deadened to know their crime.

That doesn't make it right. But to make it through—out and away—I have to endure and accept this violation, its disgrace. Preferably alone because no one can change Glen Crest, not even Abby. I can't afford my neighbor's fussing. Her concern pulls me out of the crawl space, away from being tucked into the seconds ticking by, all attention on moving one iota of time closer to seeing my Dandelion. And if I come out of the crawl space to be embraced by Abby's warm, human caring, I will crumble. I don't know if I will ever get up from the disgusting linoleum. Empathy will change nothing—certainly not Glen Crest. Its ways are as old and entrenched as the linoleum.

How many violations through open doors to rooms where other residents are hog-tied recipients of the ruthlessness that permeates this place of "rehabilitation"? Abby cannot be the only witness. What is their reason for acceptance?

Monday and the best-case scenario arrive, with one box of right-size ostomy wafers appearing on the chipped veneer of 212's dresser.

SUDDENLY, IT FEELS LIKE springtime in 212. Cell phones and their harmful emissions are banned at Glen Crest, but the dial on the clunky beige rotary gets exercised more than usual one early morning. I am making arrangements for my discharge, which is happening in mere days. Butterflies, birds, sun, and the fresh smell of growing earth are all over me and the room.

My new body is prone to falling. The bum foot is encased by a plastic brace, an ankle foot orthosis billed AFO, which holds my numb limb in place. In spite of that, I am slowly crossing floors now. *Yes!* I am walking.

Sean Sean—whose support in the PT space has been like having God giving me a hand—promises I will gain stamina once I'm home. I won't need the wheelchair at all and will only need a cane short term after I leave the gates of Glen Crest.

His words are a rare boon I lean into, never worrying if they'll hold true. I have all the reasons in the world to be full of spring and the hope of a new season.

It is time. My little girl, whose way is to express every nuance of what's running through her, is silent on her end of the phone. Her chatter is gone, and her questions are gone. She, too, has gone into a crawl space, holing herself up because she can't come home. She never begs anymore. She is just quietness—nothingness—when we speak. The awfulness of hearing that nothingness cannot be endured, and I put it into more steps—on the stairs, on the PT floor, in 212 between PT sessions. I need to get my little six-year-old home before time takes her completely.

Darkness hovers outside the dusty louvers when I awake. Things aren't right. The cot is soaked with sweat. I shiver, and the din of a noisy machine fills the room. Many gasps later, I realize it's the sound of my own breathing. Things really aren't right. It's as if my body is a lump of jelly, unable to turn over and search for the useless call button.

I need help. I am scared. Something is happening, and I don't know its name. My head, too, is jellied, and I drift in and out of its gumminess.

I sense a pink uniform entering the room. She takes a few steps toward the cot.

"I need help," I rasp. "*I'm . . . not dddoinggg well . . . fever.*" I push the words through the jelly. Then there's no more air left in me.

"Oh, just roll on your side and go to sleep." The LPN never turns on the light, never checks on the body in the bed, and only slips out of the unlit room, leaving behind the sound of begging for help. Even though my brain is jelly mush, it lets me know I've been dumped in Siberia wearing nakedness alone—a petrifying, lonely experience—and I don't know how it will end. Each chilling second is a fight for the next breath.

How often does she make this choice? How often does that pink uniform make the choice to leave someone to die?

AT SOME POINT, MORNING breaks, the shifts change, and a different nurse enters and notices 212's condition.

Within minutes, sirens sound their arrival, and I don't know which moment I am in. The room fills with EMTs, a gurney, and ER gear before an ambulance rushes down to the ICU at the nearby hospital.

Twenty-eight days no longer matter. I am in physical hell, in the ICU with double-sided pneumonia, and doctors are fighting for my continuation for an unknown number of days. I lose track of everything and only sense the excruciating fire in my chest. Yet a Viking body—even an emaciated, barely walking, malnourished version—is hard to extinguish.

Belle is finally permitted a brief visit; she appears a strained, jumbled mess next to me in the colorless linens, her trim body wearing clothes she'd normally not be caught dead in. Her hands and voice quiver, and for the first time, I see that these past months have brought hard times not just to Dandelion and me but also to the saint next door. The past days have been touch and go, she tells me—days of not being allowed inside the ICU—and she is so sorry because she thought I was doing fine. Like everyone else, she had the impression that I was cruising along and would soon be homebound.

Belle's sobs won't seize. She grabs my hands, holding them to her, as if I might otherwise disappear.

There is so much I don't say. Belle's price tag for being my savior is already too high, so I don't tell her about the Snickers meals that set me up for pneumonia. I don't tell her who the uniforms are when lights are off at Glen Crest—potential killers. I don't ask what they tell Dandelion when her mama doesn't call for days or however long it has been since my last rotary dial to Florida. The need to survive hospital, rehab, and ICU beds has made me master the skill of selectiveness.

PNEUMONIA BEATEN, I RETURN to rehab at Glen Crest, where I must pick up learning how to cane walk. It turns out that Medicare has a loophole that allows for a twenty-eight-day extension. *Oh no! Longer? I can't.* They've kept my cot vacant—a unique, considerate gesture, unless profiting from the loophole is their real motivation.

Everything changes when I check into 212 again. My body remains jelly, and the setback in the PT room is alarming. Sean Sean tells me not to worry because time is a healer. I no longer listen attentively to his advice.

The biggest change happens when I now stare at the ceiling bulb, my back against the cot's linen gloom. A spark is missing: the spark of fight—and faith. I do know that if I don't leave this godforsaken place soon, my mind will disappear. This place is not survivable. If they don't kill you physically, they will take your spirit. Yet I don't see a nearby exit. I no longer know how to get myself and my girl home.

I am going to pot, just like the rest in the corridor.

DAYS LATER, ON A March morning, I am staring open-mouthed at the nurse in my room.

"Your TB test is positive," she says rapid-fire, as if I know exactly what she's talking about. "A transporter is on its way. You're going into isolation at St. Mary's. Immediately. Get your things, ASAP."

Her back flashes out the door before I have a chance to . . . nothing. I can't speak. I can't think. What just happened is incomprehensible. Did someone do a tuberculosis test on me? A prick somewhere I wasn't let in on? Isolation . . . *for how long?*

I have just been struck from left field, an overwhelming surprise hit, and I have yet to collect myself.

Instead, I am given just enough time to grab a handful of items before I am sequestered in a dark space behind double doors, protecting the outside from the potentially infectious disease in me. Staff entering the isolation unit wear protective gear that instantaneously gets discarded after each entry and also makes them think twice before entering again. I am ordered to stay in this bleak lonesomeness, where no one comes and no one cares while waiting for more accurate testing results.

I am just a machine now—a thing that endures one more medical ordeal, that abides one more perpetration, that accepts one more procedure stripping me of any residue of power. I lie immobile in bed for hours, days, while time becomes a nonentity I have no will to resist. I say nothing, I feel nothing, and my thoughts are only dim mental waves of which I have no recollection.

Of course, the TB hoopla turns out to be a false positive. I am no better off for that. Prison isolation exists to break the spirit. I don't know about TB isolation, but its effect is the same. My spirit is just about snuffed out. Even a Viking with the best yellow flower down south to keep her going has her limits, her breaking point.

I know my next stay at Glen Crest will be my last, one way or the other.

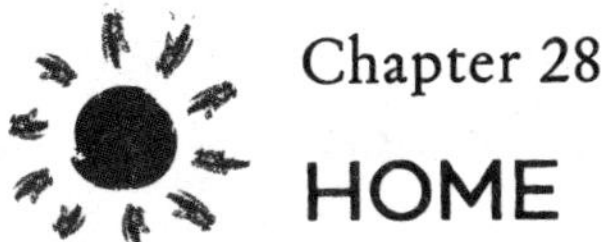

Chapter 28 HOME

Then, my release finally happens. My soul has already escaped, and now, at last, my body does, too. Straps, a wheelchair, and a corridor of hollowed-out people are left behind. I am out of Glen Crest for real. I made it, and just barely so.

Shamrocks brighten up the road home; the spirit of something Irish is in the air, and I am back in life, where small things matter. A garbage truck, stoplights, school buses, and a March morning so full of fresh air and sunlight luxuriousness that I have never encountered the likes of greet me.

I cannot grieve for the warehouse of corpses I have left behind. On this day of all green, my heart just isn't big enough to hold this ache. But the corpses are not forgotten. Their plight is not forgotten. Neither is their spiritlessness. Even years later, the stench of their withered souls and simmering human decay will tug at me, as real and heart-wrenching as the first day I was pushed through the basement entrance. They are my people, whether I want them or not. By a hair's breadth, I made it out. They didn't.

Perhaps Glen Crest will be revamped over the years, linoleum and drab rooms updated, but somewhere—despite a fine cover story—there will continue to be other Glen Crests with the same concealed, killing mercilessness that could be yours, your family, or your loved ones' destiny. But Glen Crest and its kin aren't the real problem. We are. Society. We sanction and build the ways that allow a place like Glen Crest and its uniforms to come into being.

Karla drops me off at home. She has kids to mind, so Belle is waiting at the door, full of shine and with gilded bangles dangling from ears and wrists.

With flying speed, the day is gone, and I am hobbling up the stairs to my very own bed, clad in fresh, smooth sheets bought by Belle. I dive under the covers and feel heaven has come for a visit.

HOME IS WONDERFUL. I have a brace and a bag to help me walk and defecate, though, and my new life is high-maintenance in ways not known before. There is no roaming up and down the stairs to get a glass of water or snacks. Each step is mapped out like a road trip. The Medicare-sponsored aide—reticent, wide-hipped Martha—cannot be of help because it goes against rules to fix breakfast or clean floors, so she tucks and re-tucks the sheets on my precious bed and then encloses herself in the upstairs bathroom, from which a trail of cell phone chatter leaps into the quietude of my darling home.

Being home is all that matters.

Well. Not all. Of course, it also matters that the return of my girl has been interfered with. Dandelion is not here, and she will not be coming for a while. Once more, while occupying a bed in the medical system, I've been checkmated in my own life, as if I already were a "Dementia. Bad one." This time, not by uniforms but by those who are supposed to have my back: my family.

It was my sister's initiative to stall my daughter's homecoming, and Mother Karin and Cal agreed. For his own personal reasons, Cal won't abide by my begging to have Dandelion return, although he only sees our daughter on the infrequent occasions when he stops by his sister's house. In Denmark, Mother Karin and Sallie also ignore my pleading, my need to have my girl come home now. They won't hear that Dandelion is troubled, unable to fit into a school and family life that isn't hers. They won't have it. It is only within my power to decline Martha's Medicare services and wait for Mother Karin, not Dandelion, to arrive at my sanctuary in Seaside. I must endure one more extension.

I don't fully understand my family's reason for postponing what I need most of all in the world. I want to be angry, and I am, but something else is bigger than this old feeling, and I let it go.

Mother Karin is on her way. The situation is no longer too much for her, and that's wonderful.

DAYS LATER, A BIG, black airport limo arrives, the front door swings open, and Mother Karin beams her public smile at me. "Nette, this is Reuben. Do say hello. We've been talking about Poland and how he misses his grandmother's cooking. He's going to take me back to Newark when I leave."

A nondescript driver enters and stacks Mother Karin's suitcase, bag, and fur coat in the living room. He nearly bows as Mother Karin tips him, and then it's just the two of us on the couch.

Mother Karin's smile deflates and becomes her own. "You don't look good," she says to me.

I don't mind. I don't mind anything, because my mom is here. The old anger or the new anger, the anger at her for saying things and doing things against me, is gone, and it is an unprecedented thing to be so filled with gratitude and largeness for the flaws of others that neutral is the new reaction. I hug Mother Karin and thank her for coming. Sincerely.

We have both changed. Mother Karin washes windows and runs the vacuum cleaner, just like at Halfdansvej 9, while I fit my new body and its maintenance into a routine where there is no shortage of towels and soap to handle the inevitable explosions. She is downstairs, and I am mostly upstairs, and her stay feels like a fresh way of being—harmonious. When Mother Karin asks for the car keys, I know where she wants to go because she doesn't ask me to come along. And for the first time, it's all right that she's going to the liquor store to stock up.

Mother Karin's daily drinking has been going on for years, but she is a widow now, bereft of the man she gave her heart and years to. Her breathing is also going to pot from years of cigarette smoking. I don't fight her ways; I let her drink her drink—whiskey made into a steamy tea look-alike. She cooks, we eat, we chat—carefully avoiding mentioning Magnum, whose absence is still too painful to put into words—and let each other be in the countdown to the greatest event of my life.

I am not alone in this; Mother Karin is with me, and if anyone could duplicate the tension, the longing, the anticipation going on inside me, it would be her. Something in little, willful Dandelion, who has shown up every summer and Christmas full of giggles, anger, and refusal to be told how to behave by a pointed finger and knitted brow, has opened Mother Karin up to grandmotherhood. Dandelion has made a mormor out of Mother Karin. She has done for Dandelion what she doesn't do for anyone else: She's cooked favorite dishes, played Uno until the sun's left, snuggled on the couch during movie time, and asked for kisses from her granddaughter, all with love's unwavering desire. Unlike her cousins, Dandelion has never hovered, scared, in a corner when Mormor has slammed the kitchen door, roaring something about sandy feet; she simply ignores her grandmother's outbursts. Mother Karin—Mormor—is no longer poor in kisses, and right now, she's pacing up and down the living room floor while I sit like a statue on the brown leather couch.

The plane has landed at La Guardia.

I don't breathe. I sit. I wait, though I can wait no more. Take no more. My heart refuses. Mother Karin opens the front door and steps aside. The car has arrived curbside, and Cal is on the sidewalk. Luggage emerges. Little feet move on the stairs outside—a hesitant figure in the doorway—sun-kissed hair, a miracle. Just like that. A miracle and throes, a crawl space, and three months of sheer survival are gone. She is in my arms, her face against my skin, and it is summertime in my heart. Just like that. Her little body softens into mine, and we suckle on each other's physical presence, and there is no space for words. Not yet. Maybe never.

Love purifies. Love clears. Love cleanses. That is how love works. On this day in April 2006, I am filled with the greatest cleaning action, one that overturns the darkness life dealt me during our separation.

Bliss. Just like that.

My girl is home.

DANDELION MAY BE SIX years old, but she, too, has aged. Her nails are chewed away, and the sun-kissed hair cannot hide that she has lost her shine. There is new gloom in her fine features, and the girl who firmly directed her aunt Helen and grandma to leave rather than intoxicate the New Jersey TV room and SpongeBob with their loudness is no more. Dandelion no longer cries, laughs, or chats. She has returned a quiet copy of her old self, aged in experience, shorted on childhood's blossom.

Despite our changes, our family trio builds a new routine and settles into a different kind of Seaside life.

Mother Karin and Dandelion spend a lot of time in the treehouse in the backyard in the fresh April air. Mormor makes her swing fly high, screaming glee and forgetting about bum lungs. She swoops down the slide and jumps with exuberance like another six-year-old in her best attempt to bring the sparkle in her granddaughter back.

I watch them from inside the kitchen, knowing suddenly that I have been raised by a six-year-old, someone who has mastered losing herself to play like only the precious young do. She's mastered little else; still, I am full with thankfulness for my mother, who does her best, and for my daughter, who is tucked away somewhere and anything but whole.

ONE AFTERNOON WHILE I'm resting, Dandelion begs me to go to the attic with her. She has something to show me. Her brown eyes are full of intensity, and the AFO and I brave the steep staircase. Up there, surrounded by walls painted a perfect playroom yellow, Dandelion pulls me to a corner and points to the floor. "Look, Mama."

"What's that?" I am looking at a mysterious dark pool on the worn wooden floor. It must have appeared since I last was here, months ago. I lean over and notice the wizened body of a bee, overcome by the moist darkness.

"I gave the bee honey. I didn't want it to die." Pause. "I gave it a whole big jar. But it didn't help, Mama. The honey didn't help it. It is very alone. Dead."

My daughter's voice still sounds like silver bells, though it's wobbling now, losing its clarity. And then it bursts. She crumples into the cries that have been tucked away in her for far too long. Dandelion cries at last, in my arms in the attic and in the spaces that follow. She is crying some of herself back. Crying for the motionless bee to whom she brought sustenance, the little being she couldn't help. It just lies there, not breathing. She is crying for good reason.

I silently promise my little girl that I am going to make myself so full of breath that her eyes and smile will sparkle once more. If it is the last thing I do, I will make myself rise and breathe fully.

Even darkness has its blessings.

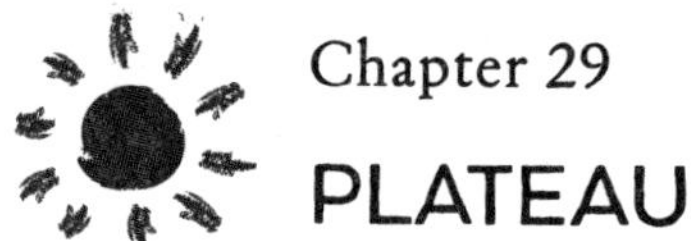

Chapter 29
PLATEAU

Danny's deep-toned voice tells me to push, and I do. I do everything Danny says.

Twice a week, I come to his office and do whatever he orders. Mother Karin has left, and we miss her. Dandelion leaves on the yellow bus each morning, and I am still finding my way with my new body.

Danny's good-natured hands remove the Velcro on the snappy ankle weights. The background noise in the PT space is National Public Radio, and Danny chats about his golden retriever and teen girls while stretching my bum foot. Danny is someone you just listen to. There is zero humbuggery in this man. He knows the human body and its marvelousness. Its intelligence. Its potential. He has been working with it for thirty-some years. He speaks with kind, firm straightforwardness. He is just my kind of man.

"If you get tired, rest. If you get sleepy, sleep. Listen to your body. No overdoing at home, okay? Listen to it, okay?"

I nod vigorously. I am one patient Danny need not push.

"We want you moving forward," he says.

"You think the doc was right?" I search Danny's all-American eyes, hungry for something I can moor my will to. He knows his trade, healing bodies. "That I shouldn't expect much improvement?"

Today is a day like any other in early spring, except it isn't. I've just been to see God.

I had an appointment with him yesterday down the LIE, exit 33. The right foot and leg may be out of an inhospitable bed, no crane or wheels needed, but truthfully, progress seems like a Danish spring hare: You think you see its white bunny tail coming toward you on a field dressed in fresh, verdant green but then it's gone—maybe altogether an illusion. The lower right leg is an atrophied stick half the size of its peer. All muscle and nerve have left. The foot droops, its bottom has lost its capacity to sense anything but burning, and the toes still resemble huge potatoes. Only the wizardry of the AFO keeps this formerly fit, toned limb in place and facilitates some sort of forward motion.

At 2:30 p.m. yesterday, I met the specialty physician whose unpronounceable area of medical expertise and decades of studying have granted him God status. As he pored over complicated tricolor curves on a printout generated by attaching electrodes to my foot, his accented English—he sounded like he'd stepped directly out of an Eastern European movie—told me things were looking very bad. In fact, "*not guuud, not guuud.*" So not good that the nerves were too damaged for repair.

I stared at the blues, yellows, and reds on the paper and their power, resting in God's hand. Then I made sound return to my voice and the office space.

It takes true mettle to go against God's judgment, even if he's a bad-looking one you hardly can understand. But I had to announce that, truly, it couldn't be that I would need the plastic brace and the sneaker ship forever.

The harsh, striking sound of God's gavel was the last din in the office. Its echo still hasn't left my mind. No improvement is to be expected, it sang, but a life dragging an AFO and huge foot along is. When I opened my eyes again, God had packed up the medical device spewing futures made from tricolor curves and left without saying goodbye.

Though Danny has never seen a bum foot like mine before, he trusts not printouts but the human body. And the body knows that where there is a will, there is always a way. *Always.*

"It's too early in the game to make predictions," he answers. "You're not even off first base yet. Let your body heal. When you heal, it heals. I'd be surprised if you didn't make improvements."

I like Danny not just because he is on my team but because he is a man with his own faith: optimism.

"Let's put on twos today, all right? Building your core is what's going to get you moving forward. Any day we can increase reps or weights is a good day."

Danny snaps on Velcro, and I lift.

Of course, I beg to differ with God, whose religion is to know what he's been schooled in, nothing else. Unlike me, he is unaware of the emerging energy medicine paradigm embraced by author Dr. Caroline Myss and others, which posits that the body isn't just a biological machine but also an energetic entity expressing our experiences, psychological stresses, and feelings with symptoms and disease. Indeed, every illness corresponds to a pattern of deep-seated emotional and psychological beliefs that have influenced specific areas of the human body. This God's training has turned him ignorant of what lies beyond medical school and is leading him to perpetuate a science of limited possibilities. He is blind to the magic powers of an individual and her body, and equally blind to the fact that whatever ails the soul *must* express in the body.

This truth I first recognized when anal pain forced me into taking frequent lavender baths, connecting me with ancient wisdom. Like a prized possession, I have carried this insight with me ever since, and have acted on it repeatedly by seeking truth. And reading Myss's bestseller has only validated and deepened my understanding of the undeniable connection between body and soul. Today, I may be hobbling on a limb that won't make any green light. Today, I may not know if my toes are touching water or fire or a car brake. Today, I may not be able to bend down and tie my shoes. All those trivial, daily leg-moving actions I used to take for granted are inabilities, feats of Grand Canyon proportions. Yet today is a good day because I put on two-pound weights for the first time, and tomorrow, I am seeing the energy medicine practitioner again—my fifth or sixth visit—to release hidden issues in my bum foot and leg. My walking will improve. The AFO and sneaker ship will be gone—because I will it.

And because God and his curves say it will not.

IMAGINE A WORLD with fewer Gods and more Dannys bringing hope and potential to those who are healing. Uniforms who nourish the formidable healing potential we all carry, our innate beat to balance ourselves. Which no curve can ever capture. And no Rx ever can replicate.

Words hold energies, intentions, truths-in-the-making. Fewer Gods and more Dannys—that's a medical revolution worth imagining.

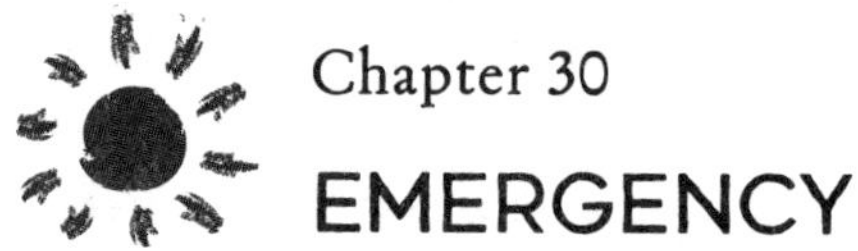

Chapter 30
EMERGENCY

I am in my bed again, but lying here feels nothing like heaven today. Snow has fallen overnight; flakes cling to the windows like angels of protection. Today marks almost 365 days since a terrible day in December 2005. Except it doesn't feel so far away. I shiver in the green linens.

Dandelion enters the bedroom; her American Girl dolls are locked in a hug, and she is brimming with chuckles. That's new. Or something old restored in a new way—and *that* is heaven.

"The dolls want more kisses!" my girl exclaims like Julie Andrews on stage, throwing her arms in the air with affect.

I move the covers aside to let Dandelion and the dolls crawl in next to me. We are once more in bed—with shivers, toys, and soon, a picnic.

That feels like another version of something old. It feels terrible.

Yesterday, I was in a place I was never supposed to meet again. Yet there I was, sweaty from pain—or perhaps sweaty from the verdict Dr. Green's fine touch on my abdomen couldn't stop. I was braving an emergency office visit.

The gastro surgeon's kind brown eyes moved away from the yellow-tinged bulge on my abdomen and looked at me. "Ms. Nilsson, it appears you have an abscess. We have two options."

Oxygen was already in short supply from the growing pressure somewhere in my gut, and now it faltered altogether. *Oh no.*

Either option was an apocalypse, even with my savior involved. How could the operation to remove the bag and restore normal defecation—a standard job, I was told—have gone so wrong? Ten days earlier, I'd been discharged, but something in me was still so very wrong. Instead of a bag, it turned out I had a festering wound.

The yellowness was a big, growing pool of pus, Dr. Green was saying, and a medical complication with two possible recourses. The personal complications of both those recourses were of such terrifying scope that my armpits wet the blue gown I wore.

In less than a second, I answered Dr. Green. My answer was an easy choice, because there was no choice. Christmas was coming, and Dandelion and I had so much to make up for. My fresh start had just been given legs, and it couldn't be stopped, not now. I could not disappear again. *We* could not disappear again.

"Option two," I whispered in the chill, sterile exam room. The lesser purgatory would have me go home right after the soaked blue gown was discarded. Home to the girl whom I'd promised to move a world for, if need be.

If Dr. Green had been a different man, he would have placed his hand on my shoulder as he told me, "Ms. Nilsson, it is going to hurt. Hurt a lot. But I will numb you as much as possible."

Perspiration and almost-tears twirled along with a sudden, frigid terror around the exam table where I was sitting. "Okay."

I shut my eyes to the tools summoned to the room in seconds: Sandra the assistant, swabs, super-size syringes, a surgical lancet, and a surgeon's kind composure.

It doesn't take long to slice someone open. Even if it felt like an eternity in Dr. Green's exam room. An eternity where the festering yellowness was lanced and everything around me stilled, everything inside me stopped, while screams wouldn't, couldn't jump out. This moment was an excruciation too great even for my soul to leave. A brutal sensation, a hurting like the kind a medieval rack used to tear limbs apart might inflict, overtook everything, and a big bang of unimaginable torture exploded in every atom of my body.

Just when I was about to faint, Dr. Green's urgent voice broke through the big bang.

"More gauze. Much more gauze. Fast."

The rack receded from the room. Dr. Green and the assistant were ministering the draining of yellowness. I drew a big inhalation, at last. So much purulence was leaving my body.

The office visit disembowelment was way worse than any terror I could have imagined. Yet it was an option I'd pick again, if need be, because this course of action allowed me to not check back into St. Mary's.

THE PURULENCE KEEPS building up, and I'm forced to return for follow-ups in the subsequent weeks. Never do I doubt that Dr. Green hopes, like I do, that the persistent yellowness is a fluke about to disappear, as if the lancet is a wand. Neither do I doubt that Dr. Green is leaving his surgeon's comfort zone by executing "option two" over and over, trying to shield me from a bed I cannot bear. But the yellowness doesn't withdraw, and twenty-four days of Christmas, a tradition vital to the Danish soul, is knocking.

This December, I had planned to make up for all we lost

last year. Instead, I am spending most days in bed or on the brown leather couch, overcome with despair and terrifying office visits. Fear sucks all my energy. I can't open a book for spiritual support or light a candle or say a prayer to connect to the spiritual realm, as I have done in the past. I can't get in the car to see the energy medicine practitioner I've been trusting to release subconscious beliefs and traumas. Foster and Kristos are on tour somewhere—Europe or South America—helping others access their issues and hidden truths. Lynn has a long wait list. I am on my own, and I have no energy to reach for my usual resources to deal with this crisis situation.

Today's been a harrowing day. This morning, the abdominal dressing covering the lancet incisions revealed not only pus but also brownness. That's a big bang of its own variety, testing the space beyond all endurance. My body still has a will of its own, and it's working against everything I'm striving for. Stool leaking from my bowels is the latest edition, and I know what the dirty dressing adds up to: a bed I cannot bear.

My body and I are still way out of balance. I am without merriment, down from the bleakness of what is to come.

When evening arrives, Dandelion skips up next to the couch. "Mama," she whispers, leaning into my ear, a pleasing breeze. "I want to show you something."

I turn and smile, waiting for my girl's revelation. It *is* Santa Claus season.

Dandelion points to her jammies, the jammies I couldn't buy for her, but someone else did last February. They're swarming with redness and Valentine hearts. "Show me, *skattepige*."

Tonight, the Julie Andrews affect is absent. Seriousness alone moves her voice. "When I was in Florida, these hearts were filled with sadness because I couldn't see you," her silver-bell sound whispers. "But now they are filled with happiness."

A whisper in your ear from a seven-year-old must be the most touching of all in this world, especially if she is your girl. Especially if you doubted her return. I throw my arms around Dandelion. I hold her tight. She is my forever blessing.

My girl is healing, and I am not.

That's when I decide it's over. I do have a choice just now. I must be greater than my circumstance, greater than my fear. Dandelion's on the right track, and I'd better join her, not thwart her return. Santa's in the Seaside air, a cat is meowing outside, and I am not in dark isolation; there are many other blessings, if I only pay attention.

In that beat, the twenty-four days of Christmas begin with sincerity. *Make my own magic.* That's the choice that follows. And with that choice, fear recedes, and energy returns.

And we do. We make our own magic, and the Danish Christmas spirit begins growing in all corners of the house. Pebernødder—tiny, crunchy, nut-shaped cookies rich in pepper and ginger—are baked and munched; gold, white, and reds are pulled from storage and hung everywhere little fingers can reach. The signature white candle decorations from my childhood with pine cones, green sprigs, and bright berries are handed out like apple pies. Each dawn reveals an overnight visit from Julemanden: A gift from Kris Kringle himself appears next to a number on the embroidered Christmas calendar, dancing with festive elves. Morfar Magnum's CD with songs of holiday spirit, reindeer, bells, and snow plays in the background, and we are two happy souls singing along.

THAT CHRISTMAS MAGIC leaves after Dr. Green informs me the CT scan has revealed an operation gone wrong. The lancet can't ever fix what's going on below the dirty dressing. Following this call, I have to summon a force greater than the perseverance of Perseverance herself to keep the merry-making up. This is done second by second; over and over, I must choose the force of joy over the alternative on the couch. Dandelion dances around like the elves, full of mirth and anticipation of the next Christmasing, never bogged down by Future's heavy hand.

As with anything, practice is what forges a new mold, what burns a fresh track in the subconscious mind. I continue choosing joy over misery, and Dandelion and I join caroling events at school and eat steamy rice pudding with melted butter and cinnamon, a seasonal treat, despite a lot of trips to the basement in another hospital where Dr. Green is on staff.

The miserable have no medicine but hope. Dr. Green has fresh hope for turning the dirty dressing around with experimental treatments.

In the morning, after Dandelion rushes to the kitchen to light the wick that burns away another number on the Christmas countdown candle, I undergo a gluing procedure amid mask-covered, blue-gowned technicians. Dr. Green is present in the chilled procedure room, watching, ordering, and checking that the gluing is done right.

For the next few days, Dandelion and I craft cards and mail them off in merry spirit; then I undergo another gluing attempt. One more basement procedure with no name. And another. The dirty dressing is unyielding, but so is Dr. Green, who conceives of more trial-and-error attempts.

In the end, all that matters is that the twenty-four days of Christmas has reached its final countdown, and I am still at home with my girl. The hearts on my girl's jammies are no longer sad, and I am merry.

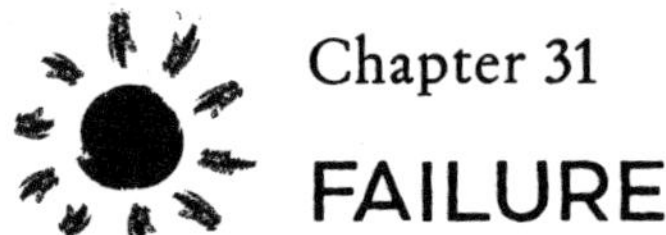

Chapter 31

FAILURE

I am waiting for the enemy. Dr. Green has sent me. He's out of rabbits and, likely, hope.

April ticks away, and the day is about to turn ever so bad. This exam room is like any other—cold, impersonal, dread dripping off the walls—in spite of its prominent address. Once more, my savior has gone beyond the call of duty and pulled strings he didn't even know he had to get Ms. Nilsson supercharging past a yearlong wait list and into this room.

God to the Gods enters. Something in the room trembles. She's fiftyish, wearing regular clothes, spunk in her eyes, and she is not one of them. She's outright personable, her smile unmistakably as wide as Sister Sallie's, stretching into the medical space and melting some of the trembling away. Her blue name tag reads "Dr. Abel," and she asks if a slew of residents may join us and if I would like anything to drink.

Mount Sinai is a very old teaching hospital, renowned internationally for its excellence, and it is the place you seek when you're out of options, up the creek, or just want the best expert advice. Dr. Abel leads Mount Sinai's Inflammatory Bowel Disease Center and is outright chief in the universe in expertise regarding what bowels can and cannot do.

She tucks the blue gown back in place, as if closing curtains on something nasty. Then God to the Gods steps away from the exam table and seeks direct eye contact—no flinching. Her strength, her expertise, her high-ranking success looks at me, its frankness not to be avoided, and I don't close my eyes.

"Only someone with your fortitude could endure this tube."

Tell me about it. Yet her comment is no compliment and it has me tearing down an imaginary track, striving to outrace the foe with a blue name tag at my heels, feeling not the least bit fortitudinous. Grief has me running, bolting. I don't want to hear what comes next. *Please.*

Just before Christmas Eve, another outpatient procedure by Dr. Green outfitted me with my very own ornament, a three-quarter-inch pipe protruding from below the navel to facilitate drainage, quite like the wastepipe at the shit factory in Frederikshavn that releases sewage into the ocean for easy elimination. For three months now, I've lived with the belly pipe inserted inside me, its sturdy plasticity rubbing against organs and bringing me to move and feel like the Tin Man. The belly pipe bursts and spews like the bag of yesteryear, equal in its cruel unpredictability, and my mind has been trained to constantly await the next purulent expulsion.

Since this pipe's placement, I have abandoned every thought of any holistic or soul-seeking healing endeavor, even though I know with all my heart that physical symptoms are covers for one's issues and that healing starts from within. The physical body and soul are a team that together creates healing, but I am merely surviving, and attending to my spirit is an impossible luxury.

The belly pipe is also Dr. Green's final attempt to give the bowel spot that won't heal a chance to heal. Rue was present the winter day Dr. Green told me in his office that we had tried all possible procedures and surgery would be the next option.

As long as I could live with the drain, so could he. Perhaps if given more time, the resection would heal. *Perhaps.*

I need more time. Much more time with my girl. That's why I am full of fortitude. That is why this situation—being a perverted, depraved, sick abomination who shoots shit through a belly pipe—is another truly-no-choice matter.

Right now, standing next to a gray wall, a slew of residents rustle their feet with restrained impatience, stretching their necks because they want a better look at a once-in-a-lifetime medical spectacle. They might as well be gawking tourists minutes away in Times Square. I get that the belly pipe is a wonder that is making their day and that they want more. This unusual medical contraption is something to put into their own personal file—witnessing, assessing, and doctoring a human bodily deviance few get to see. I abide Dr. Abel, who opens the curtain once more for their viewing. They're learning, after all.

Today is not the first time my shit-freak status has been the talk of a hospital. I was literally born in shit at Mississauga General Hospital when a hysterical Mother Karin, alone with her big belly and pressing delivery, had an enema administered but didn't make it in time to the toilet seat. On her way to relieve herself, her rectum let out an expulsion on the linoleum floor, and she slid in the brownness, both gown and pride getting smeared in her very own muck. Before a nurse managed to intervene, Mother Karin barricaded herself in the bathroom—excrement, dirty gown, and all—while filling the hospital with her screams.

Attempting to resolve this unusual delivery incident took everyone from the nurse to the director of the hospital, armed with liability waiver documents, but Mother Karin wouldn't unlock the door. Only when baby Nette started crowning did she agree to face the world in her tarred and feathered state, clueless that staff cared mostly about liability papers, not her soiled condition. That's how I came out of the womb and into a chill delivery room, unwelcomed by a young mother feeling rejected and covered in her own stool. Shit was my way into this world—my first impression and welcome, along with a large, white-coated crew of onlookers with their own agenda. Shit defined my beginning, and shit is still defining my existence today.

It's absurd the way life works, the way our beginnings shape us. Young Mother Karin's excrement accident made her feel rejected and shamed by medical people and their program, so she rejected her newborn. Now here I am, another young woman, feeling the grief and rejection of my own sorry shit and freak status. Because I am not blind to what's atop the agenda in the lineup of stares around me; their main priority isn't my welfare but their own careers.

Yesterday morning, just after waking up, I felt as if a dike burst inside; torrents of brownness rushed through into a very dirty dressing, making the pipe work overtime. Today, being here with God to the Gods, awaiting judgment on my welfare, on me and my little girl, is a world full of sorrow that I am not big enough to carry.

I look directly back into the spunk of Dr. Abel's eyes, and I hear her say:

"Nette, I don't think it's going to work. You've been on liquid nutrition for several weeks now, and the outflow is worsening. You've also tried the glue procedure twice and other failed trial attempts. The resection is irreparable."

All time leaves the room.

And then I find myself in Times Square, shooting across its bustle in my Jeep. I am going home.

I know masters when I see one. God to the Gods is one, in the field of white coats. Masters you trust, right? *Wrong.* I trust the sudden power in my heart, a power that tells me what my bowels can and cannot do. That's where true mastery comes from: listening to your heart, its unadulterated truth, even when—nay, especially when—you are in survival mode and grief or fear freezes you up. My heart power tells me my bowels can do so much more than what a Mount Sinai gavel commands it cannot, no matter how many times Dr. Abel recommends surgery to Dr. Green. I'll even help God to the Gods teach the residents a thing or two. I'll teach them a patient who says, *No!* to the story of the medical system—the story without hope, without copower.

The story of hope's potential is a wasted power that someone must claim. A slew of students are being taught that my body can only fail, a verdict of no confidence in a positive medical outcome that must be countered without flinching to halt a system gone wrong.

I drive all the way home.

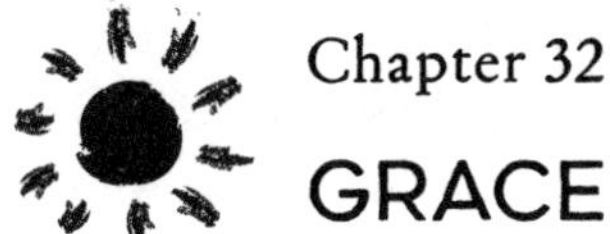

Chapter 32
GRACE

Sometimes grace gets you in destinations you never imagined.

Three days ago, I was counting kids' beachwear: Ariel . . . Belle . . . Jasmine . . .

Next, I made thirty-six Peptamen cans—my food for the coming week—fit into a suitcase, leaving room for little else.

And now we are here, in the Dominican Republic, in a nice resort picked out by Cal. Yes, Calvin. I am still fortitudinous with a belly pipe, while Cal has been a resident of this Caribbean island for some time.

During this Easter week, Brits swarm the sculpted walkways alongside white bungalows and teeming red bougainvillea. Several head toward the same spa as me. When Cal extended an offer for us to visit his new island home, alive with sunshine and beaches, the grayness of winter was hovering over Seaside, and Dandelion hadn't seen her dad in a while. I had no energy to make Eastertime at home, and agreeing to this trip came easily. That's new, and the arrangement is all good, despite having to use the wheelchair service at the airport and despite Calvin still being Calvin.

Right now, Dandelion is at the beach with her dad, and I get spa time. We are not a family, and yet, just now, we are. The warm yellowness hitting my shoulders is its own kind of nourishment, the kind that makes me look up. And grace is no accident.

I hurt. I ache. But Enis is a woman with tender hands. She reminds me of crimson hibiscus and the soothing sound of azure waves caressing the shore at dawn, like a pianist's drifting solo while the sun lifts itself off the horizon. A waft of almond oil trails her hands as they touch the misfortune of my limbs, and sweetness lingers in the dimly lit room.

Enis is a Caribbean masseuse; her silky skin is a rich caramel color, contrasting with my own pasty complexion. Her touch is gentle—careful, even—as if she is stroking a newborn's cheek. Her hands are small engines of love, softly and masterfully searching for the brick-red scars that are beginning to heal.

When Enis turns around, I notice that she has a big female behind, wide and curvaceous in her too-tight jeans. Her voluminous booty is a stark contrast to my own emaciated rear, and the bones sticking out on my body like sorrowful twigs on a tree that long ago surrendered its leaves in anticipation of winter. I'm a walking skeleton compared to Enis's fine curves. Enis exudes sultriness and youth. I don't. Enis commands the crude attention of men. I don't. She's hot, and I'm not. Not anymore. We may be the same age, but I am an old woman, hunched over, afflicted, and barely hobbling along. A freak, as you know.

"Hurt here?" Enis presses one of my toes with caution and reveals square, white teeth, evenly lined up. Another asset. She's not smiling, though, but is all presence as she delves into my body with a tender grip.

I nod, my eyes already closed. Pain is ever-present in and around my bones, though I'm not looking for any pity. I came for wafts of almond oil pressed into my skin, softening its tautness. With her wide cheekbones, smashing smile, and velvety skin, Enis could threaten any model off the runway, yet she labors in this dark room and answers to the *señora* at the front desk who checks in tourists like me who come for a lymphatic massage. At night, Enis probably leaves the resort and takes a bus that travels over bumpy, gritty roads ridden with deep potholes for an hour or two before it dumps her in a small hamlet that never would be considered a hamlet on the mainland. I bet she lives in a small shack. Yet I envy her.

"Hurt?" Enis asks again. Her hands are now touching the bottom of the crippled foot. It still droops.

I nod and cringe.

The cleansing massage is rigorous, even with a pair of hands like Enis's. It finds the atrophy, the withering-away that makes the shin look mismatched compared to its companion on the left. I sink deeper into the table's warm caress.

Moments later, Enis whispers into the spa space while her palms skim along my body, soft, soul-wise—"Accident?"

The masseuse, who has used most of her English vocabulary on me, sees into all that I am. Sees that I need to be cleansed of something that has nothing to do with organs and lymph system. Sees that *I* need to be cleansed. Cleansed of a past that is hunting my marrow and wrecking my body. That has turned me into a barren woman, disfigured and wizened long before my time, despite all my efforts to overcome it.

Then, I am struck by grace.

One sound does it. *Accident*. Sweet, hot Enis twists her tongue to break Spanish syllables into English-sounding ones. The accented sound reverberates in my head. Or rather, in my heart. *Accident*. Of course, I look like a car accident to the masseuse's dark brown eyes—the result of a freight trailer smashing a two-door sedan in a sharp turn or perhaps a nasty collision on the highway involving several speeding cars and bad brakes.

I taste the word over and over. *Accident*. It's outright delicious. I appear to be the result of an unfortunate moment on the road somewhere, not repeated trips to the hospital, rehab, and procedure room. The scars and their wounds, each with different dates and circumstances attached, are simply the result of an unlucky automobile crash that maimed its driver.

I'm an accident. That ought not to be news to me, because Mother Karin told me so: I am a creation that never should have been. They already had one daughter; another one was superfluous, simply not wanted, not between two immigrants scraping out an existence.

Enis, too, tells me I am an accident, but her loving, reverent whisper makes all the difference. In one grand swoop, I am merely a bundle of casualties, and this frees me from the crippling past that has owned my present. And my future.

The almond oil has penetrated my limp skin, mollifying dead cells into a smooth surface resembling the purity of Amish butter. Beads of sweat spring forth on Enis's forehead. A tiny fan blows the rich fragrance of nuttiness across my body, yet I don't feel the room's heat. I only feel the cleansing that the accident, shrouded in Enis's reverence, has brought me. In one word, sweet, hot Enis has granted me the pardon I have been in search of for years. Because if I am an accident Enis's way, I am also not a freak. I am *not* the unwanted baby born in shit, the newborn whose blue clothes the nurse removed because Mrs. Nilsson insisted it had a penis and she, too, was in doubt. Or the baby girl Mrs. Nilsson considered an ape. Or the tomboy with embarrassing, kinky hair. Or the hospital scarecrow. Or the belly pipe–wearing cripple-in-perpetuum sporting bodily deviances. Here in a warm spa room, I am accepted, seen, loved, and cared for under a soft touch, for being someone anyone could happen to be.

That's a destination of grace.

How do you explain this destination, this grace striking a Caribbean spa room when a masseuse by the name of Enis pours love over a decrepit body—changing a story, removing it? Healing it. I experience a sensation of goodness in all that I am, more than a trillion parts made right. This part cannot be retold justly but must be experienced. In this moment, the lame food, the AFO and shriveled leg, the belly pipe jutting out amid a bizarre tapestry of scars and barely healed holes, no longer matter. Neither do the concealed menaces lurking: the compromised heart and lungs, the terrible anemia, the severe malnutrition, the degeneration in the back, the deep-vein thrombosis, the repulsive vanilla-flavored cans of medical nutrition, the heavy-handed pain . . . the current list carries on. Grace displaces, pardons, something I have always borne, like a concealed piece of the garment even I forgot I wore: the fear of not being loved, of not being lovable, of being the baby ape that was an accident. In this instance, the fear is gone—for such is the alchemy of grace—and I stop thinking of the next catastrophe about to hit my tall, undernourished body with hurricane strength, no matter how merry I make myself be. In an unforeseeable instant, a dark, hidden spot inside me is accepted, as if brought under the glow of a Caribbean sun and melted away. There is no word wide enough to hold how it changes me—changes my outlook, changes my story's outcome—without warning. Such is grace.

A knock on the door and a quick exchange, a volley of sounds, passes between Enis and *Señora.* The next customer has arrived.

Enis squeezes a few last drops of almond oil into my skin. She moves next to my head and rests her hands on my crown, stretching out a final moment of spa peace. She is full of grace.

I leave the spa and Enis not knowing that one day in the future we will be connected in a different way. The kink in our hair, one brown and the other blonde, will turn out to share ancestral lineage. Uncle Frank—after he retires from doctoring—will find genealogy and spend his daylight hours poring over the names of my forefathers in the north, one of whom married a mulatto woman from the Caribbean and brought her to Frederikshavn. The white afro of my childhood, I will learn, has island ancestry.

That's a synchronicity of souls threaded in ways our minds cannot conceive. Beyond spa peace. Threaded by grace.

This grace is no accident. Receiving the universe's outmost favor is something I have paved the way for by befriending faith and gratitude after finding myself stuck in a version of myself I didn't know, at the biggest bash of the new millennium, and striving to redo this version for seven long years. It's called prep work, counting blessings, and having faith in all sorts of things, no matter which fear or catastrophe is lurking. One must leave a door open for grace in order for her to appear just like that. She doesn't do breaking and entering.

THE PIANIST'S DRIFTING solo has played a new day into being. The sun has risen, and I am on a walkway to the beach; thick hibiscus and bougainvillea blooms fill the warm island air. Alive with red and pink, colors and fragrances, I am going to find my girl. If anyone can see the revolution in my steps, it is her. Yesterday, grace struck, and it stayed overnight.

My feet aim for the Caribbean turquoise as if I am one of spring's first sprouts, throbbing to shoot up and out and fill the world with my refreshed, verdant appearance. The force that is spring, the earth battery that starts new life and separates us from being in storage, has gotten me good.

Suddenly, I know that there are many times when a person needs to be her own Enis. That's what I am right now. I am my own Enis. I am stroking myself full of Caribbean blushes and scents like the rich, sweet almond oil cured into my skin yesterday. I have been freed from the past, truly freed from the cover story of who I am, and that fact is transforming this now and that which is ahead.

I throb with a feeling so grand it must be the sea's own heartbeat—throb for the little girl by the beach. She saw me through 'til now. For all of her seven-year presence, right up until the moment of grace, Enis, accident, and all, she has fed me her breath. Now, she no longer needs to. I am inhaling the universe and its power. Just like that, I am becoming my own breath. Come what may—hospital beds, frowning doctors, time away—I am an accident, and grace is all around me. Even if my body doesn't look it, all is well. I know how to be now. And with that, the past turns into wisdom.

I hear happy voices and ocean sounds, and I can't wait to join in. I try increasing my speed on the walkway, but can't. I stop immediately and step next to a blooming bush for support. My hand finds a branch and grabs it. An overwhelming sensation—one that I have been avoiding for too many years—courses through my body, pushing me off-balance.

This time, I don't shut the intense sensation down but accept it. At last, I can face the grief of losing Morfar, and I allow him to appear in my heart. For thirteen years, his passing has been a dark point I have outright avoided, fearing a tidal wave of pain if I get near it. But instead of the anticipated roar of grief, I hear him, clear as day, as if I am nestled in my spot next to him on the couch, his slender arm a warm shield around me: "You," he says with his northern twang, and he pokes me in the shoulder.

I wobble and tighten my grip on the branch. A swell of emotion pulls at me, as unexpected as the grace I met yesterday, and I nearly keel over, floating into a moment so rich I can't keep my feet steady on the ground. *Morfar! You're here.* My love for him bursts open as if it has had it with being tucked away in a dark point. In a split second, I grasp how his presence, his way of always seeing me and relishing my spirit, imprinted my heart with some kind of gold, a kind that can't be erased no matter the circumstances, hardship, or pain. This precious gold has enabled me to become my own Enis. I had to find my own way, with invaluable helpers on the way, and I have now because I was built with a golden thread of worthiness, a hidden undercurrent that propels me forward through any kind of hardship, wound, or love shortage. Because Morfar's affection for me being me, when childhood shaped my personality, is built indelibly into my very essence.

In a space on the walkway that only belongs to us, I find Morfar's lapis blue eyes, and I answer, "Yes."

We guffaw, and my heart could not be any fuller. Instead of grief and pain, I find only love.

I inhale deeply, twice or more, and Morfar fades away. The warm island air sweeps against me. I stay by the bush with my hand gently on the branch, relishing the lightness inside me. People pass by with towels tucked under their arms, chatting. The moment is pure perfection.

A familiar male voice rises in the distance above the medley of resort sounds. Despite the sharpness of Calvin's pitch, I notice that the swell of love stays with me. Giggles rise inside my chest. Even in a resort filled with hundreds of people and their holiday clamor, the ocean a rushing beat in the background, Calvin makes himself heard. That's some ability. The usual annoyance I experience when his overbearing sounds fill a public arena doesn't appear today. Instead, I chuckle with newfound acceptance. Calvin didn't have a morfar. Besides, he invited me into his life years ago and recently to this Caribbean resort, and if it weren't for these invitations, I wouldn't be here by a thriving bush, empowered with the gifts of today and yesterday.

In the next moment, perhaps because my heart already has burst open with Morfar's appearance, a truth I've kept hidden from myself leaps out, and tears stream down my cheeks: On the awful day when I awoke from a coma, fighting the nurse and the facts of what had happened and also fighting for my own life, it was Calvin who sat on the chair next to the hospital bed, wringing his hands. He, of all people, showed up, and not because he had to. He showed up because he wanted to. Does that erase all the hurt he projected onto me during our time together? No—and yet, yes, in some ways, it does. Because I am changed. I appreciate now that we, two wounded people full of flaws, drew one another into our lives for many reasons, but one of them was love. Imperfect love, for sure, but love nonetheless. This recognition is a closure I need. For myself and for my daughter's sake. I am, at last, freed from an old story about Calvin and now able to tell her truthfully what I always have known but was too injured, too disempowered, to claim: *You were made from love.*

And then it is time. I wipe tears away from my face and leave the bush and the memory of the two men who shaped me and my life in ways that must have been written with a permanent pen in capital letters into my blueprint, and I head directly toward the ocean.

There she is in her Ariel swimsuit—soaked hair, a Viking frame of her own, and feet rushing in the sand toward me. "Show me, Mama. Show me." Shouts from my girl greet me above the sea's calming roar.

I leave my towel by her beach bed. Our hands grab the air, jubilant with sun and water, and then I tear off the AFO and wobble into turquoise sprays, holding my seven-year-old's palm.

Rolling waves, girly giggles, a whole lot of frisking around, and an afternoon that's just soul-happy. The way it ought to be for a seven-year-old and her mama. Because soul-happy is our nature. Lost more than once, perhaps, by a river or elsewhere, but never forgotten. Soul-happy is never forgotten.

The brace lies shipwrecked in the sand next to Brits in beach chairs with beaming red noses, though a gavel's slam told me it never would be so; it simply was not possible. And yet here I am—walking without a brace. Against all sorts of odds and gavels and cover stories, I have made it happen. I beat a system and medical Gods that believe in impossibilities.

Compassion cannot be charted and charged. Grace cannot be charted and charged. Maybe that's why healing is something the medical system truly has no feel for. My soul is no longer in the dark, appalled. By grace, it has found a way through to this blue-winged resort, rich in sea, surf, and moments just right.

The waves hammer kindly against us; we tumble, and more giggles burst; Brits turn magazine pages and order more beer. We are the grace of being ourselves, the best thing in the world, two universes released into one.

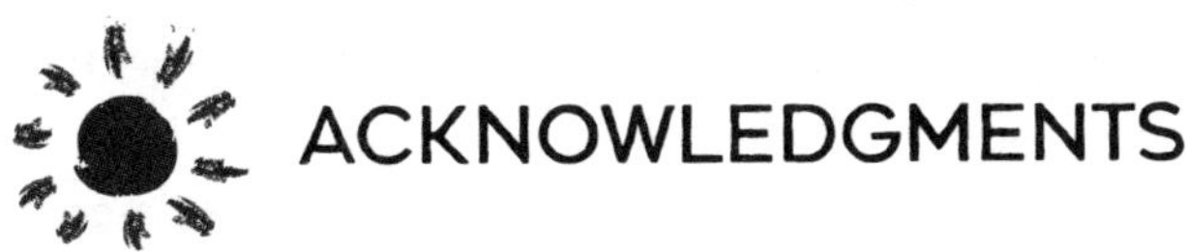

ACKNOWLEDGMENTS

I am not an expert in anything, except finding cafés that serve great cappuccinos, but I do know what being stuck in a life I never intended to live feels like. *Soul-Happy* is about the long road I took to get unstuck, find answers to my pain and distress, and return to the birthright that is ours: feeling soul-happy. Young kids know this place, and I made a promise to myself years ago that I would claim that sacred place again. That said, this book is ultimately about second chances—with myself, with my family, and with life.

Please note that my memoir is written from *my* perspective. From *my* memory, journals, recordings, emails, and files. From *my* truth.

Early on, I discovered that writing and publishing a memoir requires a community, and I have been supported in sharing this story by many exceptional and warmhearted people. There are so many individuals to express gratitude to.

The first note of thanks goes to my entire family. I traveled far to find my true self, and I could not have arrived here without the power of love and laughter and empathy that you instilled in me. It is my hope that, as reflected in my story, you feel the gratitude and love I hold for each and *every one of you.*

I'd like to express special gratitude to my deceased grandparents, whose home was my sanctuary.

To Mormor, my maternal grandmother, you left a legacy—for good reason, our family still adores you. Thank you for, in your unassuming way, being a beacon of a balanced, wholesome, spirited lifestyle—and for saying good night to the moon every evening.

To Morfar, my maternal grandfather, thank you for cherishing me.

Linda Davies, my first writing instructor and editor, deserves special thanks for mercifully reading through hundreds of pages of a diary-like manuscript and encouraging me to continue shaping my story. Thank you, Linda, for your grace, wisdom, and kindness. You made me believe in my writing abilities, and you played a significant role in helping *Soul-Happy* come to be.

To Bonnie Hearn Hill, you entered my life unexpectedly at a time when I needed a fresh set of editorial eyes assessing my manuscript. I treasure everything you taught me in our many phone conversations. Your unwavering belief in my memoir helped me trust that my book deserved to be published. Thank you!

To Brooke Warner, a profound thank-you for your visionary publishing leadership and your admirable transparency. You are changing lives by giving books like mine a trusted and inspired stable of their own.

To the women at She Writes Press, especially Shannon Green, Krissa Lagos, and Barrett Brisket, I am deeply grateful to you for handling every single detail and step with the utmost professionalism and heart. I couldn't have asked for a better support team! A special thanks to Krissa for instantly grasping my intentions and honoring my writing style; many thanks for your gentleness when proposing edits.

To my dedicated beta readers, who read my work and provided insight, cheering, and encouragement ad libitum—Annie Bachelder, Deb Rhodes, Heidi Borglum Jensen, Jodi Byers, Joseph Calderon, Rauni Siljander, Tina Laurelli,

Theresa Christensen, and Treasure Pascal—thank you! Your contributions helped make this book a reality.

To Annie Bachelder, thank you for being an ally in this lengthy writing and publishing process. Your support has meant the world to me. I love how Google matched us up many years ago.

Lynn Leclere, your gifts and wisdom opened the door to a realm I had been afraid to enter. In your hands, there is only love. Thank you.

To Foster and Kristos Perry, the two men I consider my spiritual parents—you have graced my life in mysterious, profound ways. You are true masters. I am crazy about Foster's hugs and Kristos's dry wit, and the heart and wisdom you two possess. I cherish you both.

How do you thank saints? I hold immeasurable love, gratitude, and respect for the finest two people I have ever come across: Isabelle and Rob, my beloved neighbors. You two were surely created with a special mold. Sweet, quirky, lovable Isabelle has now passed, so I extend all my thanks to you, Rob. Bless you both.

To my friend and neighbor, Anita Konfederak, thank you for everything you have done for me and my family. You are the embodiment of kindness, always lending others a hand with an easy smile and "can-do" attitude and yet never expecting anything in return. I am honored to know you.

To Cristiana Caria, a huge thank-you for supporting me in ways only you can.

To my friends Mette and Tenna, your friendship and support contribute more to my life than you will ever know. *Tak*.

To Mia, the friend I can laugh and cry with in equal measure, the friend who loves to have fun and not take anything too seriously while at the same time choosing to grow and evolve and participate in life in all its messy marvelousness—you are the finest of lionesses, and one of the great blessings of my life.

To "Dr. Green," thank you for everything you did for me, from saving my life to getting me veggies for my hospital lunch tray. There is no measure for how your humanity impacted my life at a time when "caring care" was what I needed most of all. Thank you for being a brilliant example of compassion-based health care.

To Stevi Belle, my teacher and friend, thank you for sharing your wisdom so generously with me over the years.

A hearty thanks to every medical staff who made my visit, my stay, my procedure, and my surgery better by being compassionate and kind. May your service one day become the norm.

To Sade, my musical muse since the early nineties: I continue to lean into your exquisite, soulful songs for support and self-expression. Most of all, you provided a perfect song for the chapter I could *not* write—and it turned out to be a cinch to finish once I figured that out. Thank you for your songs and your exquisiteness.

To Megan Kelly of Literary Inspired—in your capable hands, I leave all author website and other technical items, freeing me up to do what I desire most: create and write. Thank you!

Thanks to everyone who took time out of their busy schedules to read an advance copy of this book and write endorsements.

And finally, to all other dear friends and helpers, past and present—you have enriched my life in different ways. Though you are too numerous to name on this page, I hold every one of you in my heart.

To learn more about Anette and *Soul-Happy*,
visit her website at www.anettenilssonauthor.com
or scan the QR code below.

ABOUT THE AUTHOR

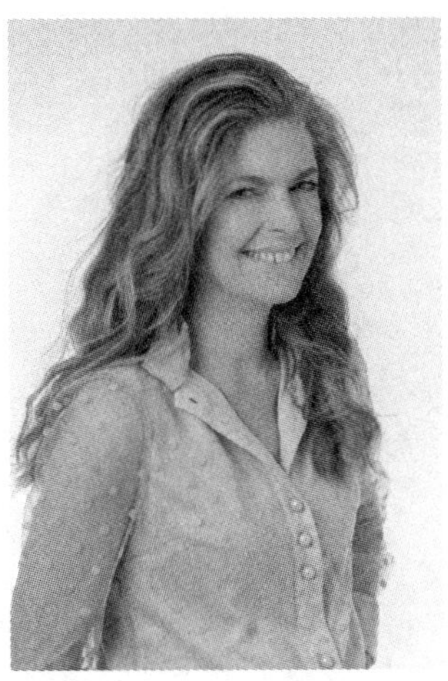

ANETTE NILSSON was raised in Denmark and spent most of her adult life in Toronto and New York. She has a dual degree in political science and criminology from the University of Toronto and studied for her MA in education at Queens College, CUNY. She founded a tech consulting firm in Minneapolis, has taught IT and English, and is the author of a children's book about three friends on an adventure with a magical raft. It is her vice to want to move to each new place she visits. Anette resides in Denmark and New York.

Looking for your next great read?

We can help!

Visit www.shewritespress.com/next-read
or scan the QR code below for a list
of our recommended titles.

She Writes Press is an award-winning
independent publishing company founded to
serve women writers everywhere.

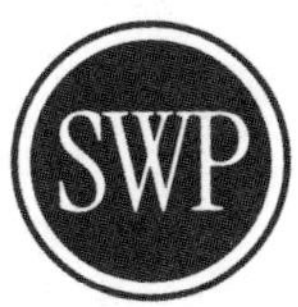